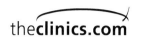

ORAL AND MAXILLOFACIAL SURGERY CLINICS
of North America

Topics in Bone and
Bone Related Disorders

MARK R. STEVENS, DDS
Guest Editor

RICHARD H. HAUG, DDS
Consulting Editor

November 2007 • Volume 19 • Number 4

SAUNDERS

An Imprint of Elsevier, Inc.
PHILADELPHIA   LONDON   TORONTO   MONTREAL   SYDNEY   TOKYO

W.B. SAUNDERS COMPANY
A Division of Elsevier Inc.

1600 John F. Kennedy Blvd., Suite 1800, Philadelphia, PA 19103-2899

http://www.oralmaxsurgery.theclinics.com

ORAL AND MAXILLOFACIAL SURGERY   Volume 19, Number 4
CLINICS OF NORTH AMERICA   ISSN 1042-3699
November 2007   ISBN-13: 978-1-4160-5101-5
Editor: John Vassallo; j.vassallo@elsevier.com   ISBN-10: 1-4160-5101-5

Oral and Maxillofacial Surgery Clinics of North America (ISSN 1042-3699) is published quarterly by Elsevier Inc., 360 Park Avenue South, New York, NY 10010-1710. Months of issue are February, May, August, and November. Business and Editorial Offices: 1600 John F. Kennedy Blvd., Suite 1800, Philadelphia, PA 19103-2899. Customer Service Office: 6277 Sea Harbor Drive, Orlando, FL 32887-4800. Periodicals postage paid at New York, NY and additional mailing offices. Subscription prices are $244.00 per year for US individuals, $358.00 per year for US institutions, $113.00 per year for US students and residents, $282.00 per year for Canadian individuals, $418.00 per year for Canadian institutions, $307.00 per year for international individuals, $418.00 per year for international institutions and $144.00 per year for Canadian and foreign students/residents. To receive student/resident rate, orders must be accompanied by name or affiliated institution, date of term, and the *signature* of program/residency coordinator on institution letterhead. Orders will be billed at individual rate until proof of status is received. Foreign air speed delivery is included in all *Clinics* subscription prices. All prices are subject to change without notice. **POSTMASTER:** Send address changes to *Oral and Maxillofacial Surgery Clinics of North America*, Elsevier Periodicals Customer Service, 6277 Sea Harbor Drive, Orlando, FL 32887-4800. **Customer Service: 1-800-654-2452 (US). From outside of the US, call 1-407-345-4000.**

Printed in the United States of America.

CONSULTING EDITOR

RICHARD H. HAUG, DDS, Professor of Oral and Maxillofacial Surgery; and Executive Associate Dean, University of Kentucky College of Dentistry, Lexington, Kentucky

GUEST EDITOR

MARK R. STEVENS, DDS, Professor and Chairman, Oral and Maxillofacial Surgery, The Medical College of Georgia, Augusta, Georgia

CONTRIBUTORS

GUILLERMO E. CHACON, DDS, Associate Professor and Residency Program Director, Department of Oral & Maxillofacial Surgery, The Ohio State University Medical Center, Columbus, Ohio

VINCENT COVIELLO, DDS, Private Practice, Germantown, Tennessee

HENRY W. FERGUSON, DMD, Associate Professor, Residency Program Director, The Medical College of Georgia, Oral and Maxillofacial Surgery, Augusta, Georgia

CARLO FERRETTI, DDS, MDent, FCD(SA)MFOS, Consultant, Division of Maxillofacial and Oral Surgery, Chris Hani Baragwanath Hospital, University of the Witwatersrand, Johannesburg, South Africa

PHILIP J. HANES, DDS, MS, Professor and Chairman, Department of Periodontics, Medical College of Georgia, School of Dentistry, Augusta, Georgia

MANOLIS HELIOTIS, MBChB, BDS, MSc, FDSRCS, FRCS, Consultant, North West London Regional Maxillofacial Unit, Northwick Park Hospital, London, United Kingdom

YI-HAO HUANG, DDS, MS, Senior Scientist, Laboratory for Applied Periodontal & Craniofacial Regeneration, Medical College of Georgia School of Dentistry, Augusta, Georgia

CARLOS M. ISALES, MD, FACP, Professor of Orthopaedic Surgery, Medicine and Cell Biology and Anatomy; and Chief, Program of Regenerative Medicine, Department of Orthopaedics, Institute of Molecular Medicine and Genetics, Medical College of Georgia, Augusta, Georgia

MARVIN F. JABERO, DDS, Resident, Department of Oral & Maxillofacial Surgery, The Ohio State University Medical Center, Columbus, Ohio

SOLON T. KAO, DDS, Assistant Professor, Oral and Maxillofacial Surgery, Medical College of Georgia School of Dentistry; and Assistant Professor, Department of Surgery, Medical College of Georgia School of Medicine, Augusta, Georgia

ROBERT E. MARX, DDS, Professor of Surgery and Chief, Division of Oral and Maxillofacial Surgery, University of Miami Miller School of Medicine, Miami, Florida

GIUSEPPE POLIMENI, DDS, MS, Senior Scientist, Laboratory for Applied Periodontal & Craniofacial Regeneration, Medical College of Georgia School of Dentistry, Augusta, Georgia

MOHAMMED QAHASH, DDS, MS, Senior Scientist, Laboratory for Applied Periodontal & Craniofacial Regeneration, Medical College of Georgia School of Dentistry, Augusta, Georgia

UGO RIPAMONTI, MD, PhD, Director, Bone Research Unit, Medical Research Council/University of the Witwatersrand, Medical School; and Professor, School of Clinical Medicine, Faculty of Health Sciences, University of the Witwatersrand, Johannesburg, South Africa

YOH SAWATARI, DDS, Assistant Professor of Clinical Surgery, Division of Oral and Maxillofacial Surgery, University of Miami Miller School of Medicine, Miami, Florida

DANIEL D. SCOTT, DMD, Oral and Maxillofacial Surgery Resident, Medical College of Georgia School of Medicine, Augusta, Georgia

MARK R. STEVENS, DDS, Professor and Chairman, Oral and Maxillofacial Surgery, The Medical College of Georgia, Augusta, Georgia

CARLOS M. UGALDE, DDS, Chief Resident, Department of Oral & Maxillofacial Surgery, The Ohio State University Medical Center, Columbus, Ohio

JOSEPH E. VAN SICKELS, DDS, Professor and Division Chief, Oral & Maxillofacial Surgery, University of Kentucky College of Dentistry, Lexington, Kentucky

ULF M.E. WIKESJÖ, DDS, DMD, PhD, Professor of Periodontics, Oral Biology, and Maxillofacial Pathology; and Director, Laboratory for Applied Periodontal & Craniofacial Regeneration, Medical College of Georgia School of Dentistry, Augusta, Georgia

CONTENTS

bisphosphonate, and the duration of use. Although intravenous bisphosphonate-induced osteonecrosis of the jaws is mostly permanent, most cases can be prevented or managed if they develop, with only a few cases requiring resection for resolution. Oral bisphosphonate-induced osteonecrosis of the jaws also can be prevented with knowledge of the risk level related to the duration of use and the C-terminal telopeptide blood test results. Most cases can be resolved with a drug holiday either spontaneously or via straightforward débridement.

characteristics of the adjacent resident bone and allows placement, osseointegration/re-osseointegration, and functional loading of endosseous implants. Clinical studies optimizing dose, delivery technologies, and conditions for stimulation of bone growth will bring about a new era in dentistry. The ability to predictably promote osteogenesis through the use of bone morphogenetic protein technologies is not far from becoming a clinical reality and will have an astounding effect on how dentistry is practiced.

FORTHCOMING ISSUES

PREVIOUS ISSUES

ELSEVIER
SAUNDERS

Oral Maxillofacial Surg Clin N Am 19 (2007) ix–x

ORAL AND
MAXILLOFACIAL
SURGERY CLINICS
of North America

Preface

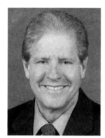

Mark R. Stevens, DDS
Guest Editor

The advances in medicine over the past several decades have come at a dazzling pace; the science of bone and its manipulation has evolved concurrently. This issue of the *Oral and Maxillofacial Surgery Clinics of North America* reviews some of those advances as they relate to oral and maxillofacial surgery and bone. I have asked each author to concentrate on "the latest updates" with regard to bone and related topics. This issue does not cover bone grafting or harvesting.

Since Urist's discovery of bone morphogenic protein, Brånemark unlocking the secrets of alloplastic compatibility of metal implantation and bone, and Ilizarov's techniques of manipulation of bone growth through distraction, continual strides and refinements in the management of bone have been ongoing. These discoveries are becoming today's clinical practice.

Advances in the understanding of bone physiology and engineering almost mirrors that of the remarkable progress in understanding the immune system secondary to the HIV/AIDS epidemic. The recapitulation of embryonic bone formation by transplanting synergistically soluble growth factors such as factor B, transforming growth factors, and superfamily and bone morphogenic/osteogenic proteins can now be used to create bone in heterotopic extraskeletal sites. Root form implants

coated with growth factors are showing exceptional results with simultaneous alveolar reconstruction.

Since Watson and Crick uncovered the DNA sequence and the subsequent mapping of the human genome, many of the specific genes and their locations responsible for genetic abnormalities in bone formation and maturation are now known. A review of the more common genetic disorders of bone and their genetic loci is discussed. With this information, genetic engineering and future correction is now a real possibility.

The nature of bone pathology has also changed. The incidence of osteoradionecrosis over the past several decades has markedly decreased. This is due to several major advances in radiation therapy. The types of radiation, its delivery and dosing, pretreatment screening, as well as improved shielding, have had an accumulative effect in minimizing radiation damage to surrounding tissue. Manipulation of bone metabolism with bisphosphonates for the prevention of bone loss and control of metastasis has also brought new dilemmas and serious undesired consequences. This family of drugs has given rise to a growing new epidemic of bisphosphonate-induced osteonecrosis of the jaw (BIONJ). New bone markers to determine risks of developing BIONJ are now being researched, as are a variety of other treatment options. Highly sensitive image technology and newer antibiotics with innovative delivery systems have continued to advance the diagnoses and management of osteomyelitis.

Advances in the areas of bone replacement by synthetic materials have evolved slower in comparison to that of growth factors. Despite the manufacturing of numerous biocompatible conductive and inductive synthetic materials for grafting and/or augmenting bony defects, predictability is still not a certainty. The article on bone substitutes is a comprehensive outline of the different types of allografts and synthetics, their specific advantages, and their appropriate applications. The management of periodontal disease has made modest strides over the past decades; however, it has not solved the problem of alveolar complex reconstruction/rejuvenation around periodontal-involved teeth. A review of the most common predictable techniques is presented. The horizon of tissue engineering seems the most promising and opportunistic. As an emerging science, it has already vastly advanced our understanding in the biochemical mechanisms of growth and differentiation of bone. As regenerative medicine progresses, new research areas and companies fabricating constructs or carriers will also emerge. Hopefully, as these new arenas form, responsible commercial and scientific endeavors will provide balanced and honest realities to practicing clinicians.

I offer my countless thanks to the many contributors who took time out of their busy lives to contribute and provide the latest information on bone as it relates to current and future practice. They are responsible for the success of this issue.

Mark R. Stevens, DDS
Oral and Maxillofacial Surgery
Medical College of Georgia
School of Dentistry Building
AD 1205A, Augusta, GA 30912, USA

E-mail address: mastevens@mail.mcg.edu

ELSEVIER
SAUNDERS

Oral Maxillofacial Surg Clin N Am 19 (2007) 455–466

ORAL AND
MAXILLOFACIAL
SURGERY CLINICS
of North America

Bone and Bone Graft Healing

Robert E. Marx, DDS

*Division of Oral and Maxillofacial Surgery, University of Miami Miller School of Medicine,
Deering Medical Plaza, 9380 SW 150th Street, Suite 190, Miami, FL 33157, USA*

Bone is unique in connective tissue healing because it heals entirely by cellular regeneration and the production of a mineral matrix rather than just collagen deposition known as scar. This article discusses the cellular, tissue, and organ levels in each of the following sections—skeletal embryology, normal bone, examples of abnormal bone, and bone graft healing—as they relate to the jaws and the craniofacial skeleton.

Pertinent embryology of the skull, facial bones, and jaws

The calvarium, facial bones, clavicle, and jaws are intramembranous bones that arise from cells that migrated from the neural crest adjacent to the notochord. These bones develop, grow, and heal by direct ossification of mesenchyme rather than from preformed cartilage. By contrast, all the other bones of the skeleton, which are referred to as the appendicular skeleton, arise from preformed cartilage by the process known as endochondral ossification. Specifically, the calvarium originates as six membrane-covered neural crest cell islands that correspond to the bilateral frontal bone segments, the bilateral parietal bone segments, and the midline occipital squamous plate and occipital bone proper separated by fontanelles [1]. The anterior fontanelle closes at approximately 1.5 years of age and becomes known as the midsagittal suture. The maxilla as well as the incus and mandible arise separately from the first pharyngeal arch. Although each arises with a central cartilage element, which in the maxilla is called the palatopterygoquadrate bar and in the mandible is called Meckle's cartilage, the cartilage

itself does not transform into bone but only serves as a scaffold on which neural crest mesenchyme transforms into bone. These cartilages involute before birth. The bones of the calvarium, facial bones, jaws, and even the clavicle have been referred to as "ectomesenchymal bone" and are thought to be embryologically similar. Bone morphogenetic protein-4 (BMP-4) also is thought to play the major role in neural crest migration orientation and actual bone morphogenesis, whereas BMP-2 plays a major role in neural crest ventralization toward the jaws and away from the calvarium but less of a role in actual bone development [2].

The conjectured and unproven importance of this embryology is that bone grafts from the calvarium are ideally suited for midface and jaw reconstruction where feasible because they are similar ectomesenchymal bones. This is reinforced by the frequent observation that calvarial block onlay grafts to the midface and jaws experience less resorption than do grafts from endochondral bones, such as the ilium or ribs. The disease of myositis ossificans also has been shown to relate to muscles that overexpress receptors for BMP-4 [2]. It has also been suggested that a recombinant human BMP-4 may be the most ideal recombinant BMP for jaw and facial bone reconstruction.

Bone as a tissue

Bone is fundamentally composed of cells, inorganic matrix, and organic matrix. The cells are hematopoietic (blood forming) and nonhematopoietic (non–blood forming) stem cells in the bone marrow, osteoblasts (of which some are endosteal osteoblasts that line the trabecular bone between the cortices (Fig. 1) and others

E-mail address: rmarx@med.miami.edu

1042-3699/07/$ - see front matter © 2007 Elsevier Inc. All rights reserved.
doi:10.1016/j.coms.2007.07.008

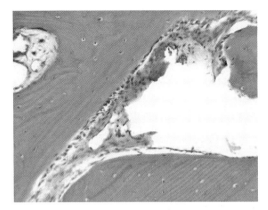

Fig. 1. Endosteal osteoblasts lining trabecular bone.

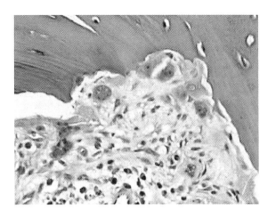

Fig. 3. Osteocytes are seen here in their lacunae. Osteoclasts are resorbing bone as multinucleated giant cells.

that line the inner surface of each cortex), and some other osteoblasts that comprise the inner or cambium layer of the periosteum (Fig. 2). Osteocytes, which are mature osteoblasts encased in a mineral matrix, and osteoclasts, which resorb bone upon stimulation and begin the bone renewal process, which is often termed "bone turnover" or "bone remodeling," are the remaining bone cells (Fig. 3). The inorganic matrix and organic matrix are combined. The basic organic component is type 1 collagen, which comprises 98.5% of the noncellular organic matrix. The inorganic matrix is nearly all hydroxyapatite. Essentially, bone matrix is mostly type 1 collagen laced with crystals of hydroxyapatite. However, there are several important noncollagen proteins in bone, namely BMP, insulin-like growth factors-1 and -2 (IGF-1 and IGF-2), sialoprotein, and osteopontin.

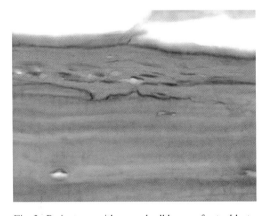

Fig. 2. Periosteum with several cell layers of osteoblasts. The inner-most layer is known as the cambium layer.

The evolutionary purpose of bone as a tissue and the skeleton as a whole is internal structural integrity, an attachment for muscles, a reservoir for hematopoietic and mesenchymal stem cells, and a main regulator of serum calcium for skeletal and cardiac muscle contraction and therefore locomotion and organ perfusion.

Bone renewal (remodeling)

The biochemistry of bone as a tissue can best be explained in the context of bone cell interactions starting with existing bone. Bone is normally inhibited from resorption by osteoprotegerin (OPG), which is a protein secreted by osteoblasts to regulate the rate of resorption as an inhibitory signal to the osteoclast (Fig. 4) [3]. As the osteoblast matures into an osteocyte it gradually loses its ability to secrete OPG and becomes vulnerable to normal osteoclastic resorption. Therefore, old bone, injured bone, and dead bone become resorbed.

Osteoclasts arise from mononuclear precursor cells of the macrophage linage in bone marrow [4]. They mature rapidly under the stimulation of macrophage colony stimulating factor and interleukin-1 and -6 (IL-1 and IL-6) and are then extruded into the circulation as quiescent nonresorbing osteoclasts because of the inhibiting influence of circulating calcitonin (Fig. 5). The osteoclast only begins active bone resorption in response to the overriding signal of circulating parathyroid hormone and locally secreted receptor activator nuclear kappa-b ligand (RANKL) [5,6]. RANKL binds to RANK receptors on the osteoclast cell membrane to initiate resorption [7]. Although RANKL is known to be secreted

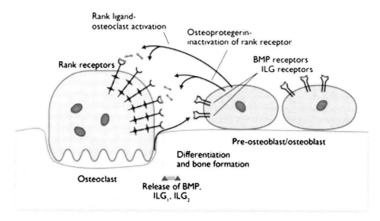

Fig. 4. Osteoblasts secrete OPG, which is a competitive receptor site binder to RANKL for the RANK receptor on osteoclasts. Its effect is to keep osteoclasts inactive and inhibit bone resorption.

by cancers to create pathologic cavities in bone [8], it is also secreted by normal osteoblasts to increase bone resorption (see Fig. 4). Normal osteoblasts also secrete OPGs as a false ligand that competes with RANKL to inhibit bone resorption by occupying the RANK receptor on the osteoclast cell membrane. This gives the osteoblast up-regulation and down-regulation control of the osteoclast and either limits the rate and amount of local bone resorption or increases it (see Fig. 4).

Osteoclast-mediated normal bone resorption begins the bone renewal/bone turnover process. The activated osteoclast adheres to a bone surface and develops a ruffled border against the bone surface as it seals the edges and forms a Howship's lacuna (Fig. 6). The osteoclast then secretes hydrochloric acid to dissolve the inorganic matrix and several collagenases to break down the organic matrix (Fig. 7). Several osteoclasts commonly work together to excavate a larger area of old bone, which is referred to as a cutting cone (Fig. 8).

Because BMP and IGF-1 and -2 are acid insoluble, they are released during bone resorption and remain as active cytokines. These released cytokines (growth and differentiation factors) bind to the cell membrane surfaces of local stem cells and somewhat to circulating stem cells to induce a differentiation into osteoblasts, and then further stimulates them to secrete osteoid. A cutting cone headed by resorbing osteoclasts and followed by a trial of osteoblasts secreting osteoid is known as a bone metabolic unit (BMU) (Fig. 9). Osteoclasts are known to live for only 14 days; newly activated osteoclasts are needed to sustain the BMU which continues for 150 to 180 days. This lifespan of the BMU is known as a sigma, and it relates that in homeostasis some bone replaces itself twice each year or at a rate of 0.5% per day.

So now bone has come full circle. The balance of bone apposition and bone resorption once again comes under the influence of the osteoblast. The young osteoblast secretes OPG as a false

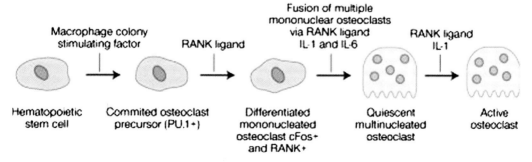

Fig. 5. Osteoclast lineage from marrow monocytes to activated osteoclasts.

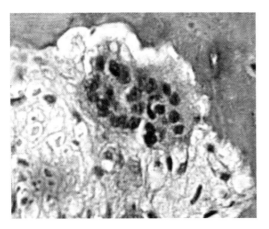

Fig. 6. Osteoclasts resorbing bone in excavation cavity known as a Howship's lacunae.

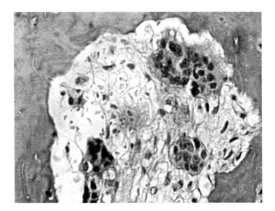

Fig. 8. Several osteoclasts work together to excavate a tunnel through bone, which is known as a cutting cone.

ligand to the RANK receptor on the osteoclast, which by competitive inhibition outpaces RANKL, so that the bone is maintained until this balance tips in the favor of RANKL by either the aging of the osteocyte (old age) or by disease so that the process begins once again. As two BMUs form new bone, they come in contact with one another and must osseointegrate to make the bone a single coalescent tissue rather than a set of mobile pieces. This is histologically seen as a cementing line (also called resting line or reversal line by some). The cementing substance is composed of sialoprotein and osteopontin, which bind two bone-forming areas together (Fig. 10). As these proteins harden by cross-linking and the collagen strands from each bone surface become incorporated into this cement substance—much in the same manner as reinforcement bars are placed into cement pillars during

highway construction—the two BMUs become bound together.

Examples of abnormal bone

The knowledge of this bone physiology helps us understand the pathology of cancer metastasis, osteoporosis, osteopetrosis, and the toxic effects of bisphosphonates on normal bone.

Cancer-induced bone resorption

Most cancers are incapable of bone resorption. Instead, they secrete RANKL to activate normal osteoclasts to resorb bone and create bony cavities into which they proliferate (Fig. 11). This is their basis for bony invasion and their metastasis to

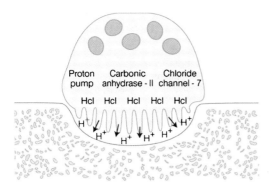

Proton pump   Carbonic anhydrase - II   Chloride channel - 7

Hcl Hcl Hcl Hcl Hcl

Fig. 7. Osteoclasts resorb bone via HCL and collagenase. They have three main mechanisms to produce hydrochloric acid.

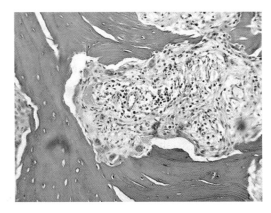

Fig. 9. A bone metabolic unit (BMU) is formed when osteoclasts resorb bone and liberate bone-inductive proteins to cause osteoblast differentiation and new bone formation.

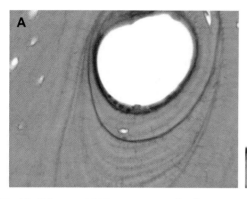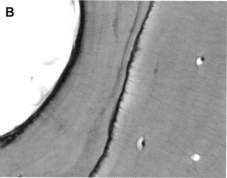

Fig. 10. (*A, B*) Low and high power cementing lines as seen here are approximately 5 μm thick and are composed of osteopontin and sialoprotein.

bone. In an effort to halt this cancer-stimulated bone resorption, the intravenous nitrogen-containing bisphosphonates pamidronate (Aredia) and zoledronate (Zometa) were synthesized. These drugs and all nitrogen-containing bisphosphonates are potently toxic to the osteoclast so as to cause their death and population depletion (Fig. 12). By doing so, the cancer cannot resorb bone and small metastatic cancer deposits are held in check. As our profession has learned, however, repetitive doses accumulate in bone, particularly bones of more active remodeling, most notably the alveolar bone of the jaws [9,10], which results in a halt to local bone renewal and osteonecrosis (Fig. 13).

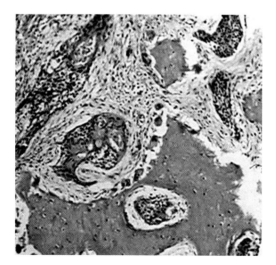

Fig. 11. Cancers resorb bone through their secretion of RANKL, which activates osteoclasts to resorb cavities in bone, into which the cancer proliferates. Here, osteoclasts are seen to be resorbing bone with the cancer cells at a distance from the bone surface.

Osteoporosis and bisphosphonates

In a similar effort to slow or halt age- and menopause-related bone resorption leading to osteoporosis, the oral bisphosphonates residronate (Actonel), alendronate (Fosamax), and ibandronate (Boniva) have been used. Their toxic effects on the osteoclast are designed to retain existing bone and allow it to increase its mineralization as measured by bone density tests and prevent osteoporosis-related fractures [11,12]. Toxicity to the osteoclast prevents resorption, which is needed to renew bone; therefore, old and more brittle bone accumulates over the years. Although they initially increase the strength of bone by further mineralization, over many years the unrenewed bone becomes more brittle, which limits its fracture prevention [13,14] and increases the risk for osteonecrosis in the jaws [15].

Osteopetrosis

Nearly identical to the pathophysiology of bisphosphonate-induced osteonecrosis is the disease of osteopetrosis. This disease of eight genetic variants, all of which render the osteoclast nonfunctional or absent, also results in necrotic bone in the jaws caused by reduced or absent bone renewal (Fig. 14). Toward the other extreme, overfunction of the osteoclast—as seen in untreated primary hyperparathyroidism—results in resorption cavities known as brown tumors and in hypercalcemia, which results in depolarized nerves and muscles causing mental confusion, abdominal pains, constipation, and weakness, the classic symptoms of primary hyperparathyroidism.

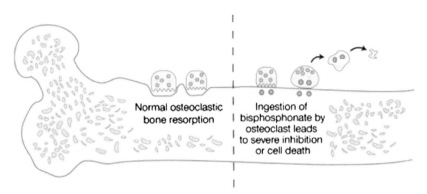

Fig. 12. Bisphosphonates cause rapid osteoclastic death by inhibiting enzymes in the mevalonate branch pathways which prevents bone renewal.

The structure of bone

The histology of bone begins with Haversian systems, which are the trademark of mature bone. Haversian systems are concentric rings of interconnecting osteocytes surrounding a Haversian canal (Fig. 15). Haversian canals are channels through which arterioles, venules, and lymphatics pass. The bony surface of the canal is lined by endosteal osteoblasts, which usually can be seen to have formed a ring of osteoid against the mature bone. Haversian canals are connected at right angles to other Haversian canals by similar but smaller diameter canals, known as a Volkmann canal. Because Haversian systems are concentric circles, they do not geometrically join. Instead, they are joined by mature bone not organized into Haversian systems but organized with lamellar bone and joined to the Haversian system by a cementing line. This area is known as interstitial lamella (Fig. 16).

In long bones, most of the shaft is composed of cortical bone organized into Haversian systems and interstitial lamella. The inner cortical surface is lined by endosteal osteoblasts and the outer cortical surface by periosteal osteoblasts. The bone marrow in the mid-shaft is mostly cellular marrow without much stroma. The adult marrow in the proximal and distant ends of long bones, the vertebrae, the pelvic bones, and craniofacial skeleton is trabecular bone with interconnections. In between, hematopoietic marrow and stem cells reside but are replaced with fibro-fatty marrow as an individual ages. Each trabecula is lined by endosteal osteoblasts and contains osteoid and lamellar bone, some of which may be organized into Haversian systems.

The importance of this knowledge is the recognition that mature bone is viable, vascular, and yet more mineral dense (Fig. 17). This type of bone results in the best primary stability for dental implants. Immature bone can be recognized

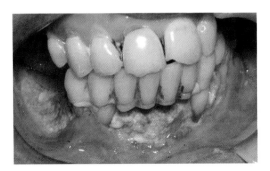

Fig. 13. Bisphosphonate-induced osteonecrosis of the jaws.

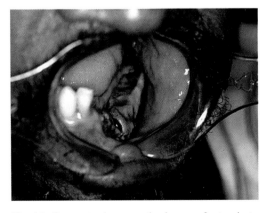

Fig. 14. Osteopetrosis, a genetic absence of osteoclasts, produces exposed necrotic bone in the jaws identical to bisphosphonate-induced osteonecrosis.

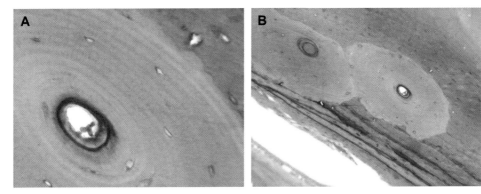

Fig. 15. (*A*) Haversian canal and Haversian system in mature bone. (*B*) Haversian canal and Haversian systems together with interstitial lamella.

histologically as much more cellular, with plump osteocytes in larger lacuna and little or no lamellar architecture (Fig. 18).

Mechanism of bone regeneration and healing

Bone grafts of any type can only regenerate bone through three possible mechanisms: direct osteogenesis, osteoconduction, and osteoinduction. Grafts may develop bone from one, two, or all three of these mechanisms to varying degrees.

Direct osteogenesis

Direct osteogenesis is the formation of osteoid by osteoblasts. Osteogenesis may occur in children without any grafting and has been termed "spontaneous osteogenesis." In these cases, the bone forms from the surrounding periosteum and from the endosteum of adjacent bone. Osteogenesis from a bone graft is often termed "transplanted osteogenesis." In these cases, numerous surviving endosteal osteoblasts—mainly from cancellous marrow because of its extended surface area and marrow stem cells—are the cellular sources of new bone formation. Autogenous cancellous marrow grafts are examples of direct transplanted osteogenesis, which migrates through the blood clot of the wound.

Osteoconduction

Osteoconduction is the formation of new bone from adjacent bone or from periosteum through a matrix that acts as a scaffold. In these cases, the matrix must bind the cell adhesion molecules fibrin, fibronectin, and vitronectin or consist of collagen itself. The natural healing of a tooth socket is an example of osteoconduction, as is

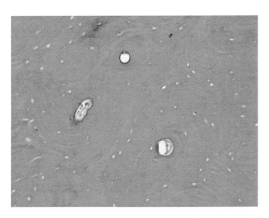

Fig. 16. Lamellar bone between Haversian systems is termed interstitial lamella.

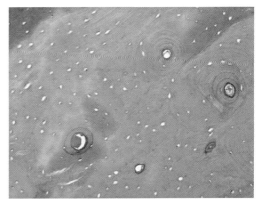

Fig. 17. Mature bone has lamellar architecture, Haversian systems, and a greater mineral density.

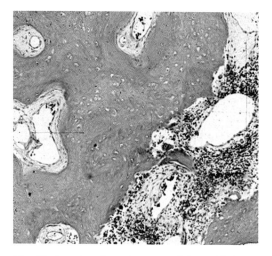

Fig. 18. Immature bone is more cellular, with larger lacunae and sparse or lamellar architecture.

a sinus augmentation graft using a nonviable graft material.

Osteoinduction

Osteoinduction is the formation of bone by the biochemical transformation and stimulation of stem cells into bone-producing cells. BMP, whether endogenous or exogenous, is the best-known bone-inducing agent.

Autogenous bone graft healing

Bone grafts harvested from the craniofacial skeleton versus bone graft harvested from the axial skeleton

The jaws, facial bones, and calvarium arise from embryonic stem cells from neural crest origin. There is a common notion that embryologically derived similar bone grafts from the calvarium perform better than bone grafts from embryologically dissimilar bone grafts harvested from long bones. Although this notion is not confirmed, experienced surgeons who have accomplished both types of grafts have noted that calvarial block grafts to the jaws experience less resorption and volume loss than similar block grafts from the ilium or ribs. This occurrence may be caused by the similarity in the residing stem cells in each bone or to similar architecture. It also may be caused by diploic vascular channels in calvarial bone that evolved to vent heat from the human brain. This competing theory postulates that this greater number of vascular channels

contains more endosteal osteoblasts and stem cells for bone regeneration while promoting an earlier revascularization. In either case, calvarial bone is preferred for grafting the midface, nasal area, and orbits and is used for larger sized maxillary and mandibular ridge augmentations where possible and practical to harvest (Figs. 19–21).

Healing and incorporation of nonvascularized block bone grafts

The mechanisms of healing and incorporation of autogenous block bone grafts are universal regardless of the donor site. The rate of this healing and the amount of final bone formation vary with the donor site, however, and depend on several other factors. The most important factors are the amount of cellular marrow transplanted with the bone graft, the vascularity of the tissue bed, and the attainment of graft stability.

The osteocytes within these grafts die off because of their encasement in a mineral matrix and disruption of their delicate canalicular blood supply. New bone is formed by osteogenesis as a result of surviving endosteal osteoblasts and marrow stem cells, which are few in block grafts, and by osteoinduction from the release of BMP and IGF-1 and -2 as the mineral matrix is resorbed and by osteoconduction through the framework of the graft itself. Block bone grafts form new bone, mostly by osteoinduction and osteoconduction from the adjacent bone margins and much less through direct osteogenesis from surviving osteocompetent cells. This is why larger block grafts form less bone and experience a reduction in their volume when used as onlay grafts. It is also why in

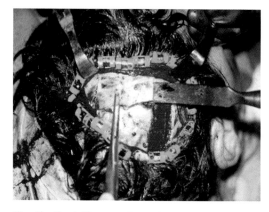

Fig. 19. Cranial bone grafts are best harvested from the parietal bone area because of a greater thickness of bone between the outer and inner table in that area.

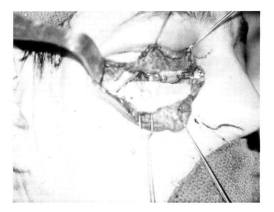

Fig. 20. Cranial bone has a contour similar to the mid-face and orbital areas and is similar to intramembranous bone.

larger mandibular continuity defects block grafts are noted to show bone regeneration at each resection margin, which tapers to the center, where a residual defect may continue (Fig. 22).

Healing and incorporation of vascularized block grafts

Block grafts on a vascular pedicle, such as a free microvascular fibula, transfer preformed mature bone. In this case, the composite of mature osteocytes, periosteum, and mineral matrix can be transferred in a viable state. Conceptually this would seem the ideal graft and is embraced by many surgeons who are not as familiar with jaw morphology, function, and the need for denture wearing as oral and maxillofacial surgeons. The problem with such preformed bone is more practical than biologic. That is, the fibula is far too small and too straight to be an adequate jaw reconstruction, particularly for the mandible. A fibula is only 10 to 12 mm in height, which is the size of each person's index finger. Placed next to a mandible, the size discrepancy becomes readily apparent. To curve such a straight and brittle cortical bone about the arch form of the mandible also requires two osteotomies. At best, it only reconstructs a small broken jaw, which is not ideal (Fig. 23).

The healing of this type of graft to the host bone is identical to fracture healing, which is via the proliferation of endosteal osteoblasts and periosteal osteoblasts through the fibrin and fibronectin of the blood clot between the bone ends. This process begins with the degranulation of platelets, which cause the migration, differentiation, and stimulation to form a bony callus. The initial internal and external callus first

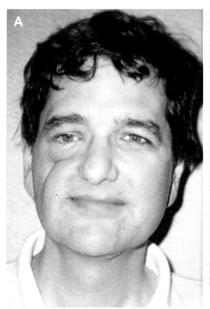
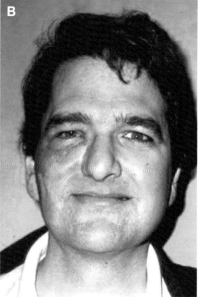

Fig. 21. (*A*) Cancer-related defect before cranial bone grafting. (*B*) Improved contour gained by a cranial bone graft. (*Adapted from* Marx RE, Stern D. Oral and maxillofacial pathology: a rationale for diagnosis and treatment. Hanover Park (IL): Quintessence; 2002. p. 819; with permission.)

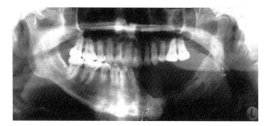

Fig. 22. A nonvascularized block bone graft often results in a deficient volume and resorption, particularly in the center, because the new bone formation arises mainly via osteoconduction from each bone margin.

consists of osteoid that unites the graft to the host bone and then undergoes a gradual resorption and replacement by new bone, which remodels the callus into a mature bony union.

Autogenous cancellous cellular marrow graft healing

Autogenous cancellous cellular marrow grafts are the most common grafts used by oral and maxillofacial surgeons and represent the most predictable outcome. Their value resides in the transplantation of more endosteal osteoblasts and marrow stem cells (osteocompetent cells) than any other graft. Their mechanism of healing—whether used in a maxillary alveolar cleft, a sinus augmentation, or a continuity defect of the mandible—is the same. It begins with the initial survival of the transplanted osteocompetent cells. These cells are open to the local environment and survive by oxygen and nutritional diffusion (plasmatic circulation) until the graft becomes revascularized by capillary ingrowth. Mature osteocytes do not survive the transplantation. Their mineral matrix is resorbed later when revascularization allows osteoclasts to enter the area.

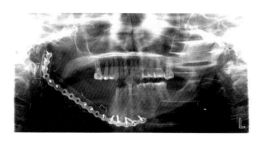

Fig. 23. Microvascular fibulas represent a poor mandibular reconstruction because they are too small and too straight.

In the first week of a cancellous cellular marrow graft, platelets regulate the bone regeneration by their degranulation and secretion of seven growth factors: the three isomeres of platelet-derived growth factor (PDGFaa, PDGFbb, PDGFab), transforming growth factor-beta 1 and 2, vascular endothelial growth factor, and epithelial growth factor (Fig. 24). These growth factors are chemotactic, mitogenic, and angiogenic. As early as the third day, capillaries are seen to penetrate into the graft and the osteocompetent cells are seen to undergo a proliferation. By the seventh day, the platelets are exhausted and contribute little more to healing but are replaced by the macrophage, which was attracted to the graft by its initial hypoxic state and the chemoattraction from the platelet effects. The macrophage continues to secrete the same or similar growth factors until the graft is fully revascularized, which occurs between 14 and 21 days.

Once the graft begins revascularization—especially when it is completed—the oxygen and nutrients it affords allows the osteocompetent cells to synthesize and secrete osteoid. This process begins at approximately 2 weeks and continues to approximately 6 to 8 weeks. Once such revascularization occurs, osteoclasts arrive from the circulation and resorb the original mineral matrix and liberate BMP and IGF-1 and -2, which begins the maturation of the graft. As the osteoid is resorbed and new osteoblasts are induced, the newly forming bone is under function. The new bone is formed in accordance with this function and tends to be less cellular and more mineral and contains lamellar architecture (Fig. 25). This process continues from approximately the sixth week throughout the lifetime of the graft but is 90% mature by 6 months. The first 2 weeks of a cancellous cellular marrow graft involve cytokine secretion and intense cellular proliferation. The period from week 2 to week 8 involves osteoid formation. The period after 8 weeks is one of resorption—new bone apposition remodeling into a mature more mineralized bone (Fig. 26).

The clinical relevance of this mechanism of healing of each graft type relates to the general choice and expectation of the graft. Nonvascularized onlay block grafts from the ilium should be oversized to compensate for their expected volume reduction of up to 30%. Although they can be used successfully to reconstruct smaller continuity defects, they are best limited to defects 3 cm or smaller in younger, nonradiated patients in whom

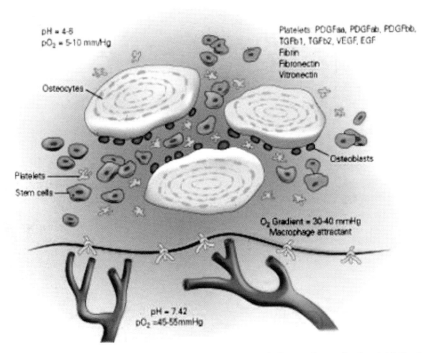

Fig. 24. A cancellous cellular marrow graft is directed by the growth factors from platelets initially then by macrophages, which cause capillary ingrowth and osteoprogenitor cell proliferation.

sufficient osteocompetent cells remain in the host bone or periosteum to bridge the defect by osteoconduction. Nonvascularized calvarial grafts are well suited for orbital, nasal, maxillary, and mandibular onlay grafts because of their embryologic similarity, which seems to confer a lesser volume reduction than other donor sites, and to their contour similarity. The amount of donor bone is limited and mostly cortical, however,

which makes this site impractical for continuity defects, many sinus augmentations, and most alveolar clefts.

Vascularized block grafts are reasonable as an immediate stabilization graft to restore continuity and facial form. Their inadequate size and lack of morphologic similarity to the jaws makes them unsuitable for a definitive mandibular reconstruction, however. Cancellous cellular marrow grafts are best used in larger defects and in situations in which their particulate nature can be contained, such as alveolar clefts, sinus augmentations, and continuity defects. Their advantages are that they

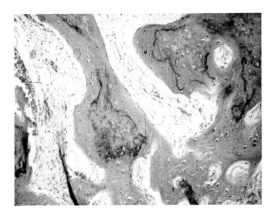

Fig. 25. Once a cancellous cellular graft becomes revascularized, osteoid is synthesized which then remodels into mature bone.

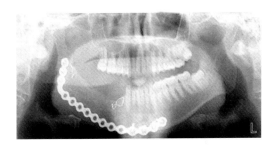

Fig. 26. The outcomes of cancellous cellular marrow grafts provide the best results related to bone height, width, and functional ability.

can be sculpted into a more ideal jaw contour, height, and width and have the least dimensional change. The bone that regenerates is active remodeling bone that responds well to functional loading. They readily support denture wearing and rehabilitation with dental implants.

Summary

Modern oral and maxillofacial surgeons are well advised to learn the details of skeletal embryology, bone physiology, bone structure, and different bone graft healing mechanisms. This knowledge will help clinicians to understand the numerous bone pathologies that require treatment and make the best selection of grafting approaches for each patient's needs.

References

[1] Larsen WJ, editor. Human embryology. 3rd edition. Development of the head and neck. Philadelphia: Churchill Livingstone; 2001. p. 358–71.

[2] Larsen WJ, editor. Human embryology. 3rd edition. The third week. Philadelphia: Churchill Livingstone; 2001. p. 75–6.

[3] Carda C, Silvestrini G, Gomez de Ferraris ME, et al. Osteoprotegerin (OPG) and RANKL expression and distribution in developing human craniomandibular joint. Tissue Cell 2005;37:207–55.

[4] Xing L, Schwarz EM, Boyce BF. Osteoclast precursors, RANK/RANKL, and immunology. Immunol Rev 2005;208:19–29.

[5] Feng X. RANKing intracellular signaling in osteoclasts. IUBMB Life 2005;57:389–95.

[6] Kaji H, Kanatani M, Sugimoto T, et al. Stations modulate the levels of osteoprotegerin/receptor activator of NF kappa B ligand mRNA in mouse bone cell cultures. Horm Metab Res 2005;37: 589–92.

[7] Kostenuck PJ. Osteoprotegerin and RANKL regulate bone resorption, density, geometry, and strength. Curr Opin Pharmacol 2005;5:618–25.

[8] Wada T, Nakashima T, Hiroshi N, et al. RANKL-RANK signaling in osteoclastogenesis and bone disease. Trends Mol Med 2006;12:17–25.

[9] Dixon RB, Truhin ND, Garetto LP. Bone turnover in elderly canine mandible and tibia [abstract 2579] J Dent Res 1997;76:336.

[10] Marx RE, editor. Oral and intravenous bisphosphonate-induced osteonecrosis of the jaws: history, etiology, prevention, and treatment. Chicago: Quintessence Publ; 2006. p. 24–6.

[11] Reginster J, Minne HW, Soresen OH, et al. Randomized trial of the effects of residronate on vertebral fractures in women with established postmenopausal osteoporosis. Osteoporos Int 2000;11: 83–91.

[12] Black DM, Thompson DE, Bauer DC, et al. Fracture risk reduction with alendronate in women with osteoporosis: the fracture intervention trial. J Clin Endocrinol Metab 2000;85:4118–25.

[13] Bone HG, Hosking D, Devogelaer JP, et al. Ten years experience with alendronate for osteoporosis in post menopausal women. N Engl J Med 2004; 350:1189–97.

[14] Black DM, Schwartz AV, Ensrud KE, et al. Effects of continuing or stopping alendronate after 5 years of treatment: the Fracture Intervention Trial Long-term Extension (FLEX): a randomized trial. JAMA 2006;296:2927–38.

[15] Marx RE, Cillo JE, Ulloa JJ. Oral bisphosphonate induced osteonecrosis: risk factors, prediction of risk using serum CTX testing, prevention, and treatment. J Oral Max Fac Surg, in press.

ELSEVIER
SAUNDERS

Oral Maxillofacial Surg Clin N Am 19 (2007) 467–474

ORAL AND
MAXILLOFACIAL
SURGERY CLINICS
of North America

Genetic Disorders and Bone Affecting the Craniofacial Skeleton

Guillermo E. Chacon, DDS*, Carlos M. Ugalde, DDS, Marvin F. Jabero, DDS

Department of Oral & Maxillofacial Surgery, The Ohio State University Medical Center, 305 West 12th Avenue, P.O. Box 182357, Columbus, OH 43218-2357, USA

Genetic disorders of bone that affect the craniofacial skeleton are individually rare; however, they have significant clinical relevance because of their overall frequency. These disorders include several that result in derangement of growth, development, and differentiation of the face and skull. The clinical severity differs greatly among individual patients, ranging from minor handicaps to death in the neonatal period. Traditionally these disorders have been divided into dysostoses (defined as malformation of individual bones or groups of bones) and osteochondrodysplasias (defined as disorders of chondro-osseous tissues) [1]. The complexity of these alterations has been known for some time. Although single entities have been described since the nineteenth century or the first part of the twentieth century, most entities we know currently have been delineated much more recently [2]. This progress has provided us with more insights into the genes that control normal skeletal development. To date, approximately 300 different types of skeletal disorders have been identified; however, only a few have a significant number of cases reported in the literature. For this reason and because of the limitations of time and space, we limit our discussion to the seven most common disorders in this group. For practical purposes we also leave out of this discussion the craniofacial disorders that involve skeletal physiognomy.

Fibrous dysplasia (McCune-Albright syndrome)

Fibrous dysplasia is an uncommon, noninherited genetic bone disorder of unknown origin. This condition is commonly found in children aged 3 to 15 years and can affect any bone of the musculoskeletal system (Fig. 1A–C). The genetic mutation is found on the guanine nucleotide binding protein gene (GNSA1) located on the 20q13.2 chromosome and can be categorized into three groups: (1) monostotic, which involves one bone, (2) polyostotic, which involves more than one bone, or (3) a form known as McCune-Albright syndrome, which involves the skin and endocrine system. An additional form is known as craniofacial dysplasia, which affects bones that are limited to the craniofacial complex [3–5]. Clinical symptoms include—but are not limited to—difficulty walking, pain, fractures, and bony disfigurement.

Fibrous dysplasia has been linked to multiple endocrine dysfunctions, including precocious puberty, hyperthyroidism, growth hormone excess, hyperprolactemia, and hypercortisolism. The most common clinical manifestation other than bone dysfunction is the presence of skin lesions known as café au lait spots, which are found in nearly 50% of the polyostotic cases. These skin lesions manifest secondarily to the excessive production of melanin in the basal skin layer.

Radiographic diagnosis is typically visualized using plain films. Severe cases that include the spine, cranial bases, and mid-face may require the use of CT scanning to better visualize the involvement of bony changes, however. This disease can affect any bone but is more commonly found in long bones, ribs, spine, and the craniofacial complex [6].

* Corresponding author.
E-mail address: chacon.4@osu.edu (G.E. Chacon).

1042-3699/07/$ - see front matter © 2007 Elsevier Inc. All rights reserved.
doi:10.1016/j.coms.2007.08.001

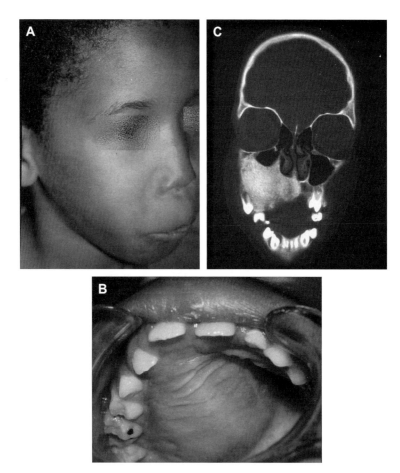

Fig. 1. An 11-year-old male patient shows clinical signs of fibrous dysplasia. (*A*) Facial view shows enlargement of the right malar bone. (*B*) Intraoral view shows involvement of the palate on the ipsilateral side. (*C*) Coronal cut of the patient's CT scan shows the classic "ground glass" appearance of the involved osseous structures.

Fibrous dysplasia of the maxillofacial complex most commonly involves the maxilla more than the mandible. Clinical signs include painless expansion of bone and tooth displacement. Radiographic evaluation usually demonstrates mixed radiolucent and radiopaque lesions with a classic presentation of "ground glass" opacity without clearly defined borders. The bony expansion may cause nerve and blood vessel compression with special concern for the optic nerve. These lesions can mimic other diseases, such as osteomyelitis and Paget's disease, and require a biopsy and histopathologic confirmation of fibrous dysplasia. Histologically these lesions demonstrate irregularly shaped trabeculae of woven bone within a fibrous stroma [4,7,8].

The treatment of fibrous dysplasia is only indicated when symptoms persist or cosmetics secondary to psychosocial factors are a major concern. The optimal treatment time is best obtained later in life when an individual has reached young adulthood because this disease seems to decrease in its activity toward the end of the second and beginning of the third decades of life. When expansion has appeared quiescent, the idea of surgical intervention can be introduced. The treatment of choice in these patients is cosmetic recontouring [9]. Patients must be advised that regrowth can occur up to 50% of the time, especially in younger individuals.

In recent years, conservative treatment of fibrous dysplasia with oral and intravenous bisphosphonate therapy has shown some promising results. Zacharin and O'Sullivan [10] ran an open trial of pamidronate treatment in five children and four young adults with polyostotic fibrous dysplasia associated with McCune-Albright syndrome to assess clinical response, bone turnover, and cardiovascular status over a 2-year period. They found this therapy to be effective in controlling disease progression and it showed improvement in bone pain, mobility, and quality of life. In a similar but longer term study, Chapurlat and colleagues [11] sought predictors of response to treatment with the use of intravenous pamidronate in 58 patients (41 adults and 17 patients younger than 18 years of age). They found that this therapy was associated with substantially decreased pain, diminished levels of biochemical markers of bone turnover, and improved radiologic aspect in approximately half of the patients treated. Although the therapy was considered safe, no clinical or biologic predictors were established. These findings were supported in a similar study by Kos and colleagues [12].

A case report from Nippon Medical School in Tokyo found similar clinical and radiographic evidence with the use of oral bisphosphonate alendronate [13]. With recent findings regarding bisphosphonate-induced bone necrosis, the question that immediately arises is what would happen if patients required surgery. With bone healing already compromised by their disease and the added effect of this new treatment modality, are these patients at a higher risk for complications? We believe that currently it may be premature to jump to such conclusions, but we certainly must be cautious when dealing with these individuals.

Malignant transformation of fibrous dysplasia is rare, with a frequency of less than 1%, and has been reported sparingly in the literature. The most common transformation is among the class of sarcomas. Treatment for these malignances remains controversial [14,15].

Osteogenesis imperfecta

Osteogenesis imperfecta is an inherited autosomal dominant genetic disorder that affects up to 50,000 people in the United States and may be found in 1:8000 individuals [5]. This disorder has been termed "brittle bone" disease because of the increased fragility of bone resulting in bony fractures under normal load. It is the most common type of inherited bone disorder. Osteogenesis imperfecta is characterized by injury to formation and maturation of collagen. Three genes are typically associated this disease: COLIA I gene located on chromosome 17, COLIA II gene located on chromosome 7, and the recently identified CRTAP gene located on chromosome 3 [16,17]. Osteogenesis imperfecta affects multiple aspects of the human body, including the development of bone, cartilage, dentin, skin, and sclera. There are at least four major types of osteogenesis imperfecta: types I, II, III, and IV.

Type I is the most common and is typically categorized by autosomal dominant inheritance. Patients usually develop fractures in the second or third decades of life and develop blue sclera and deafness as they age [5]. Type II is the most severe form of all types of osteogenesis imperfecta and affects 1:20,000 to 60,000 infants [17]. Patients with type II typically fracture bones during delivery, and death occurs before the first year of life [18]. This form is found to be both autosomal dominant and recessive. Type III is the most severe form that is associated with surviving patients who have osteogenesis imperfecta. Patients with type III develop the most severe forms of bone fragility, and most patients die during childhood as a result of cardiopulmonary complications from kyphoscoliosis. Bony deformities of the limbs may lead to altered function and mobility. Type IV is the second most common of the types and displays mild to moderate bone fragility. This type is similar to type I but has a higher incidence of fractures developing in childhood.

Osteogenesis imperfecta has an effect on the formation of dentin in primary and permanent dentitions. The primary dentition is more often affected than the permanent dentition, however. The affected dentin is part of a process known as dentinogenesis imperfecta, which subdivides each type of osteogenesis imperfecta. Some patients have no clinical or radiographic evidence of dentinal involvement, whereas other patients have a varying degree of change in dentin formation. Clinical findings include discoloration of the crowns that varies from opalescent to gray to brown to yellow. Patients with malformed dentin are at higher risk of dental attrition, fractures, and loss of vertical dimension [19]. It is important that these individuals seek dental care at an early age to help maintain appropriate dental and skeletal growth. Radiographically, dentinogenesis imperfecta is suggested by bulbous anatomic crowns, cervical constriction, and pulp chamber and canal obliteration.

There is no specific treatment for osteogenesis imperfecta; however, the importance of seeking dental care at an early age can help prevent skeletal and dental malformations. Prevention and treatment of fractures remain major issues for patients who have osteogenesis imperfecta. For this reason, implementation of different therapies geared toward preventing fractures has been attempted with a certain degree of success. In 1996, Landsmeer-Beker and colleagues [20] reported on the use of the bisphosphonate olpadronate for the treatment of this condition over a 5- to 7-year period. Their study suggested that long-term continuous administration of the drug to patients with osteogenesis imperfecta and vertebral deformities was effective. This finding was established by looking at radiographs that showed a tendency for restoration of normal vertebral shape and increased calcification of the long bones. Other studies have reported on the use of intravenous pamidronate for this purpose [21–23]. Their combined findings are consistent with the previously referenced study. Probably the most valuable observation was the decrease in the incidence of fractures found in the treatment groups.

It is important to remember that the great variability in disease can result in mild clinical manifestations or death in utero. Treatment is dictated by the severity of each patient's degree of involvement.

Osteopetrosis (Albers-Schöenberg syndrome)

Osteopetrosis is a hereditary bone disease characterized by abnormal bone remodeling caused by a deficiency of bone resorption that results from failure of production and function of osteoclasts [24]. It was first reported by Albers-Schöenberg in 1904 [25]. The abnormality in bone physiology combined with continuous bone formation leads to thickening of the cortical bone and sclerosis of the cancellous portion. The manifestations associated with this syndrome are pathologic fractures, cranial nerve palsies, anemia, facial deformities, developmental anomalies of teeth, and osteomyelitis. The prevalence of osteopetrosis is low at 1:100,000 to 1:500,000 [5].

Three different types of osteopetrosis have been identified clearly and reported in the literature: infantile malignant autosomal recessive osteopetrosis, intermediate autosomal recessive osteopetrosis, and autosomal dominant osteopetrosis (adult benign osteopetrosis).

Infantile malignant autosomal recessive osteopetrosis

The initial presentation is considered the most severe form of osteopetrosis. Usually diagnosed during the first month of life, this type is associated with pathologic fractures, failure to thrive, frequent respiratory infections, and head and neck or bony infections. Lethargy, small stature, and hepatosplenomegaly are also associated with this form of osteopetrosis. Patients affected by this condition also present with facial deformities, such as macrocephaly, hypertelorism, and frontal bossing. The abnormal resorption process can cause narrowing of the skull foramina, which results in compression of cranial nerves and causes blindness, deafness, and facial paralysis. This form of osteopetrosis can cause death during the first decade of life. Anemia also can be present secondary to the encroachment of the sclerotic bone on the marrow spaces.

Intermediate autosomal recessive osteopetrosis

This unusual presentation of osteopetrosis is similar to the infantile malignant type but appears in a milder expression. Affected patients survive into adulthood with some considerable disabilities.

Autosomal dominant osteopetrosis (adult benign osteopetrosis)

Also considered adult osteopetrosis, this type can present with few or no symptoms. Life expectancy is usually not altered in this presentation. Two types of variations have been described according to the radiologic presentation, both of which have in common a generalized sclerosis. Type I consists of a cranial sclerosis and thickening around the calvarium. In type II, the sclerosis is limited to the cranial base with an almost normal calvarium. Fracture and osteomyelitis secondary to dental extraction are the most common risks associated with this presentation of osteopetrosis. Histologic examination shows different patterns of abnormal endosteal bone formation in cancellous spaces.

Treatment of osteopetrosis consists of stimulating osteoclasts or providing an alternative source of osteoclasts [26]. Bone marrow transplant is the only hope for treating infantile malignant osteopetrosis. Corticosteroids and parathyroid hormone have been used to stimulate bone resorption and treat anemia by an increase in hematopoiesis. Limited intake of calcium and vitamin D can stimulate the production of osteoclasts [27]. Human γ-1b interferon can enhance bone resorption and increase hematopoiesis and leukocyte function in patients who have osteopetrosis [28]. Osteomyelitis of the jaws can happen because of the impaired function of white cells and poor vascular supply. The most common site is the mandible, but it can affect the maxilla [29,30]. Treatment of the osteomyelitic condition of the jaws includes incision and drainage, saucerization, sequestrectomy, and extraction of teeth in the affected area. Jaw resection and hyperbaric oxygen therapy are the only successful methods of treatment for more involved cases.

Cleidocranial dysplasia

Cleidocranial dysplasia, formerly known as cleidocranial dysostosis, is an autosomal dominant skeletal dysplasia that results from a defect in the CBFA1 gene of chromosome 6p21. This disease is characterized by abnormal clavicles, patent sutures and fontanelles, supernumerary teeth, and other skeletal changes [31]. Early diagnosis of cleidocranial dysplasia is difficult because craniofacial abnormalities become evident during adolescence. Most cases present with hypoplastic clavicles and, in some instances, with unilateral or bilateral absence of the clavicles. In some cases, patients can approximate their shoulders in front of the chest. Short stature, hypertelorism, broad nose, and frontal bossing are clinical features found in these patients. Narrow, high, arched palate, cleft palate, prolonged exfoliation of the primary dentition, and unerupted supernumerary teeth are common intraoral findings. Young individuals have normal jaw proportions and morphology but because of delayed or lack of eruption of permanent teeth may experience short lower face height and mandibular prognathism as they grow [32].

There is no specific treatment for cleidocranial dysplasia. Early diagnosis and interdisciplinary management are important in the management of this disease. Serial extractions and orthodontic extrusion of permanent teeth can prevent abnormal jaw relationships. Full-mouth extractions with denture fabrication are other modalities of treatment.

Cherubism

Cherubism is a rare genetic disease of the maxilla and mandible that results in a painless swelling of one or both of these entities. Its clinical characteristic is reminiscent of cherubs displayed in Renaissance paintings. This disease is described as an autosomal dominant nonneoplastic disease mapped to the 4p16 chromosome [33]. This condition is generally inherited, but cases of nonfamilial origination have been documented [34,35].

Cherubism usually manifests before the age of 6, and patients typically present with painless bilateral mandibular and maxillary mandibular expansion. This clinical feature produces the cherub-like appearance. Some cases involve the inferior orbital rim and orbital floor, which results in scleral show and an upward gaze of the eyes. An intraoral examination may reveal clinically missing teeth, widened alveolar ridges, and tooth displacement. Radiographically, patients typically have multilocular radiolucent lesions of the posterior mandible consistent with the bilateral mandibular expansion clinically (Fig. 2) [36,37]. Histologically these lesions are similar to giant cell granulomas, with a large volume of vascular fibrous connective tissue containing a variable number of focal giant cells [33,38]. Perivascular eosinophilic cuffing is commonly present.

Early treatment of cherubism is limited to assisting dental development and addressing specific concerns with family regarding physical appearance. These lesions are typically self-limiting, and regression is seen after puberty. If physical appearance remains an issue, treatment can be more aggressive in the third and fourth decades of life, when cosmetic recontouring is the treatment of choice.

Familial gigantiform cementoma

Gigantiform cementoblastoma is an uncommon autosomal true dental tumor. This term has been used in the past to describe florid-osseous dysplasia; currently the term should be reserved to describe this rare hereditary disorder. This disorder consists of a slow-growing, multifocal/multiquadrant, expansile lesion that involves the jaws. Radiographic examination resembles cemento osseous dysplasia. The initial phase of the disease is characterized by radiolucencies in the periapical regions. As the lesion matures it acquires a mixed radiolucent/radiopaque appearance as it replaces normal bone. A mature familial gigantiform cementoma presents as a multiple, circumscribed, lobular, and expansile lesion with a mixed radiographic appearance that crosses the midline. The lesion continues to mature until it becomes predominately sclerotic with a thin radiolucency around its circumference. Elevated alkaline phosphatase levels with subsequent improvement after

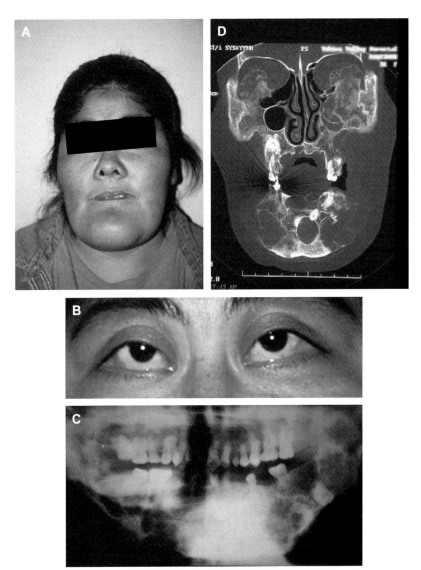

Fig. 2. A 31-year-old female patient diagnosed with cherubism. (*A*) Notice the enlarged mandible, bilateral malar prominences, and increased scleral show. (*B*) Classic ocular findings associated with cherubism. Notice the relative upward rotation of the globes as a result of abnormal tissue invading the orbits. (*C*) Panoramic radiograph shows large bony and dental involvement. (*D*) Coronal cut of the patient's CT scan shows the severity of her condition.

surgical removal of the lesion have been reported [39].

Histologically, familial gigantiform cementoma is indistinguishable from cemento-osseous dysplasia. The lesion consists of fibroblastic tissue proliferations with variable degrees of cellularity intermixed with cemental deposits and limited bone formation [40]. Treatments performed before the sclerotic phase consist of shave-down surgical procedures but are not usually successful because of the rapid growth of the disease. Attempts to

perform partial resection during the sclerotic phase can lead to sequestration of the affected bone [5]. Extensive resection of the tumor with reconstruction is recommended and has been reported with good aesthetic and functional results [40].

Gardner syndrome

Gardner syndrome is a rare autosomal dominant disease in which chromosome 5 (5q21) has been mapped as the responsible gene. This gene is also known as the adenomatous polyposis locus [41]. The disease is characterized by gastrointestinal tumors, multiple osteomas, dental abnormalities, and skin and other soft tissue tumors. The prevalence of Gardner syndrome varies from 1:8300 to 1:16,000 live births [5].

Gastrointestinal polyps have been reported to undergo malignant transformation, and their early identification is vital. Osteomas consist of single or multifocal proliferations of compact or cancellous bone in a periosteal or endosteal location that can vary greatly in size [42]. The osteomas can occur in the mandible, maxilla, sinuses, and long bones. In some instances, large osteomas of the mandible, particularly in the condylar region, can cause limited mouth opening [43]. Dental abnormalities include odontomas, supernumerary teeth, and dental impactions. Epidermoid cysts and desmoid tumors can be found in the face, scalp, and extremities.

Treatment of the cutaneous manifestations depends on the symptoms, cosmetic nature, and location of the lesions found. The major concerns regarding Gardner syndrome are the high rate of transformation of gastrointestinal polyps into invasive adenocarcinomas in 100% of the cases [44]. Prophylactic colectomy is recommended once the diagnosis has been confirmed [45].

Summary

Genetic disorders of bone constitute a large number of alterations approaching almost 300 types. Because of the limitations of this article we focused our discussion on the most common diseases in this group, which at the same time are the most clinically significant because of their incidence and degree of involvement of the craniofacial skeleton.

References

[1] Kornak U, Mundlos S. Genetic disorders of the skeleton: a developmental approach. Am J Hum Genet 2003;73:447–74.

[2] Superti-Furga A, Bonafe L, Rimoin DL. Molecular-pathologic classification of genetic disorders of the skeleton. Am J Med Genet 2001;106:282–93.

[3] Cohen MM Jr. The new bone biology: pathologic, molecular, and clinical correlates. Am J Med Genet 2006;140(23):2646–70.

[4] Cohen MM Jr, Howell R. Etiology of fibrous dysplasia and McCune-Albright syndrome. Int J Oral Maxillofac Surg 1999;28(5):366–71.

[5] Neville BW, Damm DD, Allen CM, et al. Bone Pathology. In: Neville BW, Damm DD, Allen CM, editors. Oral and maxillofacial pathology. 2nd edition. Philadelphia: WB Saunders; 2002. p. 533–87.

[6] Leet A, Chebli C, Kushner H, et al. Fracture incidence in polyostotic fibrous dysplasia and the McCune-Albright syndrome. J Bone Miner Res 2004;19(4):571–7.

[7] Reymond J, Podsiadlo M, Wyskiel M. [Fibrous dysplasia situated in maxilla: diagnostic and treatment difficulties illustrated with case report]. Otolaryngol Pol 2006;60(1):79–84 [in Polish].

[8] Yetiser S, Gonul E, Tosun F, et al. Monostotic craniofacial fibrous dysplasia: the Turkish experience. J Craniofac Surg 2006;17(1):62–7.

[9] Ozek C, Gundogan H, Bilkay U, et al. Craniomaxillofacial fibrous dysplasia. J Craniofac Surg 2002; 13(3):382–9.

[10] Zacharin M, O'Sullivan M. Intravenous pamidronate treatment of polyostotic fibrous dysplasia associated with McCune Albright syndrome. J Pediatr 2000;137:403–9.

[11] Chapurlat RD, Hugueny P, Delmas PD, et al. Treatment of fibrous dysplasia of bone with intravenous pamidronate: long-term effectiveness and evaluation of predictors of response treatment. Bone 2004;35: 235–42.

[12] Kos M, Luczak K, Godzinski J, et al. Treatment of monostotic fibrous dysplasia with pamidronate. J Craniomaxillofac Surg 2004;32:10–5.

[13] Kitagawa Y, Tamai K, Ito H. Oral alendronate treatment for polyostotic fibrous dysplasia: a case report. J Orthop Sci 2004;9:521–5.

[14] Hoshi M, Matsumoto S, Manabe J, et al. Malignant change secondary to fibrous dysplasia. Int J Clin Oncol 2006;11(3):229–35.

[15] Ruggieri P, Sim F, Bond J, et al. Malignancies in fibrous dysplasia. Cancer Cythopathology 1994; 73(5):1411–24.

[16] Barnes A, Chang W, Morello R, et al. Deficiency of cartilage-associated protein in recessive lethal osteogenesis imperfecta. N Engl J Med 2006;355(26): 2757–64.

[17] Primorac D, Rowe D, Mottes M, et al. Osteogenesis imperfecta at the beginning of bone and joint decade. Croat Med J 2001;42(4):393–415.

[18] Byers P, Krakow D, Nunes M, et al. Genetic evaluation of suspected osteogenesis imperfecta (OI). Genet Med 2006;8(6):383–8.

[19] O'Connell A, Marini J. Evaluation of oral problems in an osteogenesis imperfecta population. Oral Surg Oral Med Oral Pathol Oral Radiol Endod 1999; 87(2):189–96.

[20] Landsmeer-Beker EA, Massa GG, Maaswinkel-Mooy PD, et al. Treatment of osteogenesis imperfecta with the bisphosphonate olpadronate (dimethylaminohydroxypropylidene bisphophonate). Eur J Pediatr 1997;156:792–4.

[21] DiMigelo LA, Ford L, McClintock C, et al. Intravenous pamidronate treatment of children under 36 months of age with osteogenesis imperfecta. Bone 2004;35:1038–45.

[22] Letocha AD, Cintas HL, Troendle JF, et al. Controlled trial of pamidronate in children with types III and IV osteogenesis imperfecta confirms vertebral gains but not short-term functional improvement. J Bone Miner Res 2005;20:977–86.

[23] Falk MJ, Heeger S, Lynch KA, et al. Intravenous bisphosphonate therapy in children with osteogenesis imperfecta. Pediatrics 2003;111:573–8.

[24] Helfrich M, Aronson D, Everts V, et al. Morphologic features of bone in human osteopetrosis. Bone 1991;12(6):411–9.

[25] David BB, Martin RB. Errors in bone remodeling: toward a unified theory of metabolic bone disease. Am J Anat 1989;186:186–216.

[26] Kocher MS, Kasser JR. Osteopetrosis. Am J Orthop 2003;32(5):222–8.

[27] Mohn A, Capanna R, Delli Pizzi C, et al. Autosomal malignant osteopetrosis: from diagnosis to therapy. Minerva Pediatr 2004;56(1):115–8.

[28] Key LL Jr, Rodriguiz RM, Willi SM, et al. Long-term treatment of osteopetrosis with recombinant human interferon gamma. N Engl J Med 1995; 332(24):1594–9.

[29] Bakeman RJ, Abdelsayed RA, Sutley SH, et al. Osteopetrosis: a review of the literature and report of a case complicated by osteomyelitis of the mandible. J Oral Maxillofac Surg 1998;56(10):1209–13.

[30] Barry CP, Ryan CD, Stassen LF. Osteomyelitis of the maxilla secondary to osteopetrosis: a report of 2 cases in sisters. J Oral Maxillofac Surg 2007;65(1):144–7.

[31] Furuuchi T, Kochi S, Sasano T, et al. Morphologic characteristics of masseter muscle in cleidocranial dysplasia: a report of 3 cases. Oral Surg Oral Med Oral Pathol Oral Radiol Endod 2005;99(2):185–90.

[32] Ishii K, Nielsen IL, Vargervik K. Characteristics of jaw growth in cleidocranial dysplasia. Cleft Palate Craniofac J 1998;35(2):161–6.

[33] Meng X, Yu S, Yu G. Clinicopathologic study of 24 cases of cherubism. Int J Oral Maxillofac Surg 2005; 34(4):350–6.

[34] Mangion J, Rahman N, Edkins S, et al. The gene for cherubism maps to chromosome 4p16.3. Am J Hum Genet 1999;65(1):151–7.

[35] Silva GC, Gomez RS, Vieira TC, et al. Cherubism: long-term follow-up of 2 patients in whom it regressed without treatment. Br J Oral Maxillofac Surg 2006;45(7):567–70.

[36] Penarrocha M, Bonet J, Minguez J, et al. Cherubism: a clinical, radiographic, and histopathologic comparison of 7 cases. J Oral Maxillofac Surg 2006;64(6):924–30.

[37] Pulse C, Moses M, Greenman D, et al. Cherubism: case reports and literature review. Dent Today 2001;20(11):100–3.

[38] Kaugars G, Niamtu J 3rd, Svirsky J. Cherubism: diagnosis, treatment, and comparison with central giant cell granulomas and giant cell tumors. Oral Surg Oral Med Oral Pathol 1992;73(3): 369–74.

[39] Finical SJ, Kane WJ, Clay RP, et al. Familial gigantiform cementoma. Plast Reconstr Surg 1999;103(3): 949–54.

[40] Abdelsayed RA, Eversole LR, Singh BS, et al. Gigantiform cementoma: clinicopathologic presentation of 3 cases. Oral Surg Oral Med Oral Pathol Oral Radiol Endod 2001;91(4):438–44.

[41] Toure G. Contribution of maxillofacial signs in the diagnosis of Gardner syndrome. Rev Stomatol Chir Maxillofac 2004;105(3):177–81.

[42] Baykul T, Heybeli N, Oyar O, et al. Multiple huge osteomas of the mandible causing disfigurement related with Gardner's syndrome: case report. Auris Nasus Larynx 2003;30(4):447–51.

[43] Lew D, DeWitt A, Hicks RJ, et al. Osteomas of the condyle associated with Gardner's syndrome causing limited mandibular movement. J Oral Maxillofac Surg 1999;57(8):1004–9.

[44] Losacco T, Punzo C, Santacroce L. Gardner syndrome: clinical and epidemiologic up to date. Clin Ter 2005;156(6):267–71.

[45] Fotiadis C, Tsekouras DK, Antonakis P, et al. Gardner's syndrome: a case report and review of the literature. World J Gastroenterol 2005;11(34): 5408–11.

Role of the Oral and Maxillofacial Surgeon in the Diagnosis and Treatment of Patients with Osteoporosis

Carlos M. Isales, MD, FACP

Department of Orthopaedics, Institute of Molecular Medicine and Genetics, Medical College of Georgia, CB-2803, 1120 15th Street, Augusta, GA 30912, USA

The United States population is aging. If you are a man and reach age 65, your average life expectancy is an additional 16.8 years; if you are a woman, it is 19.8 years. The number of Americans aged 65 and older is expected to increase from the roughly 12% (or approximately one out of every eight persons) of the population in the year 2004 to approximately 15.4% in 2020 and to approximately 20% in 2030 [1]. Although 66% of patients younger than age 65 (18–64 years old) considered their health as either excellent or very good, this was true for only 36.7% of the older (over 65) patients [1]. Clinicians will be faced with an increasingly older population of patients, with an increasing prevalence of chronic health problems.

Common chronic health conditions in the elderly population include high blood pressure, arthritis, heart disease, cancer, diabetes, and osteoporosis. It is currently estimated that 44 million Americans over the age of 50 (55% of this population) have osteoporosis. It is also estimated that this number will increase to 61 million patients (80% women and 20% men) by the year 2020. Morbidity associated with osteoporosis, or low bone mass, is mainly caused by the increased risk of fractures. It is estimated that one out of every two women and one out of every four men over the age of 50 will have a fracture. This figure represents 1.5 million osteoporosis-related fractures/year at a cost of $18 billion.

Because of the increasing prevalence of osteoporosis in the aging population, it is important for oral surgeons to be aware of this condition for several reasons: (1) Oral health frequently reflects systemic diseases, and calcium loss in the teeth may mirror systemic mineral losses in the skeleton. Chronic health conditions, such as osteoporosis, also may affect surgical outcomes. (2) Because low bone mass itself usually does not produce any symptoms, osteoporosis may not be diagnosed until a patient presents with a fracture. Early diagnosis could significantly reduce fracture-associated morbidity and mortality. The role of dental radiographs in the diagnosis of osteoporosis is discussed later in this article. (3) In the past, therapies of osteoporosis were limited to hormonal replacement therapy and fluoride. Recently, there has been a proliferation of new therapies for osteoporosis that may affect dental health. In particular, the association between bisphosphonate use and osteonecrosis of the jaw is of concern. It is important that oral surgeons be aware of the medications a patient is using for the treatment of osteoporosis before initiating any procedure.

Definition of osteoporosis

Although the definition of osteoporosis seems to be intuitively obvious (less bone than normal), bone is a complex tissue with mineral (calcium-phosphate or hydroxyapatite) and proteinaceous (mainly collagen type I) components. It is this dual composition that provides bone with structural strength and flexibility. At the same time, this dual makeup makes it possible to have bones

Dr. Isales' work is supported in part by funding from the National Institutes of Health (R01DK058680).

E-mail address: cisales@mcg.edu

with a normal mineral component but increased risk of fracture or bones with a low mineral component with no increased risk of fracture [2].

The World Health Organization functionally defined osteoporosis based on bone density measurements using dual energy x-ray absorptiometry (DEXA or DXA). According to this definition, a bone density measurement at the femoral neck that is more than 2.5 standard deviations below the peak bone mass (T-score) is considered to be osteoporotic [3]. This definition takes into account only the amount of mineral present in bone without regard to other factors that might predispose to bone fragility and consequent fractures, however. Low bone density itself can account for less than half of the fractures that occur. These other factors, besides bone density, that predispose to fractures have been termed "bone quality." Having had a previous vertebral compression fracture is a stronger predictor of fracture risk than bone mineral density measurements alone. In patients with a T-score on DXA of more than −2, the fracture risk was four- to six-fold more than control patients. In patients with one vertebral compression fracture, the risk for a second vertebral fracture was fivefold greater, whereas the presence of two or more vertebral compression fractures increased the risk for additional fractures to 12-fold higher.

The combination of low bone mass and existing vertebral compression fracture was actually the best risk predictor, however, with these patients having a more than 75-fold higher risk for additional vertebral compression fractures [4]. The highest fracture risk seems to be within the first year of the first vertebral compression fracture [5]. In addition to the history of previous fracture, age seems to be an important risk factor. Studies have shown that even at identical bone density measurements, the risk for a fracture in an 85-year-old patient is much higher than that of a 45-year-old patient [2]. Partly in response to the recognition that bone density measurements are not the only important risk factors for the development of fractures a National Institutes of Health consensus conference was organized in the year 2000 and defined osteoporosis as "skeletal disorder characterized by compromised bone strength predisposing a person to an increased risk of fracture" [6]. The World Health Organization also is in the process of developing new guidelines for relative risk assessment, and other factors besides bone density measurements (eg, age) will be included in these revised guidelines.

Pathophysiology of osteoporosis

The two most common causes of osteoporosis are estrogen loss in women (menopause) and age-related loss, although there are multiple potential

---

Box 1. Risk factors for and causes of osteoporosis

Genetic
  White or Asian female gender
  Positive family history for
    osteoporosis or fracture
  Connective tissue disorders
    (osteogenesis imperfecta, Marfan
    syndrome, homocystinuria)
Behavioral and environmental
  Increased age
  Poor nutrition (low calcium intake, low
    vitamin D intake or lack of sun
    exposure, high caffeine intake)
  Eating disorders (anorexia, bulimia)
  Alcohol abuse
  Tobacco abuse
  Thin or small frame
  Inactivity or immobilization
  Prior history of fracture
Metabolic and hormonal
  Hypogonadism (low testosterone or
    estrogen)
  Endocrine diseases (Cushing's
    syndrome, primary
    hyperparathyroidism,
    hyperthyroidism, acromegaly,
    diabetes mellitus)
Medications
  Corticosteroids
  Chemotherapeutic agents
  Anticonvulsants
  Heparin
  Lithium
  Gonadotropin releasing hormone
    agonists
Malignancy or chronic illness
  Any chronic inflammatory state
    (including rheumatoid arthritis and
    AIDS)
  Cancer (multiple myeloma, leukemia,
    lymphoma, metastatic
    malignancies)
  Gastrointestinal or malabsorptive
    syndromes (celiac sprue or bariatric
    surgery)

causes of bone loss (Box 1). In the past, osteoporosis was generally divided into two types. Type I osteoporosis was secondary to estrogen loss, and type II osteoporosis was secondary to aging. Currently, these terms are used less commonly because it is clear that bone loss is a complex process not easily divided into those two categories.

Net bone mass is the result of the balance between bone formation (mediated by osteoblasts) and bone breakdown (mediated by osteoclasts). Until the age of 20 to 25 this balance favors bone accrual. In women, bone mass remains relatively stable until menopause (although changes in estrogen levels may begin up to 5 years before menopause), at which time a decrease in estrogen levels leads to a phase of rapid bone loss. This phase of rapid bone loss progresses over several years (4–8) and then continues at a lower but steady rate [7]. Examining bone density at the femoral neck specifically, age-related bone loss is approximately 0.5%/year. Bone loss at the femoral neck related to drops in estrogen levels (peri-menopausal/menopausal) is approximately 5.3% (for the 3 years before the last menses and 4 years after the last menses). In contrast, bone loss at the spine seems to be exclusively secondary to estrogen deprivation [8].

Estrogen has multiple effects on bone, with direct effects on osteoblast and osteoclast function. Osteoblasts and osteoclasts express estrogen receptors-alpha and -beta [4,9], although estrogen receptor-alpha seems to mediate the major estrogen effects on bone [10]. Levels of numerous hormones/cytokines are altered by estrogen, including interleukin-6 (IL-6), IL-1, IL-11, IL-7, tumor necrosis factor alpha, macrophage colony stimulating factor, receptor for activated NFkβ ligand, and osteoprotegrin [10,11]. More recently, nitric oxide was implicated in mediating estrogen effects on osteoclasts [9]. Several reports also highlighted the effects of estrogen on the immune system. It is recognized that estrogen can modulate T-lymphocyte differentiation through an IL-7–dependent mechanism [12,13]. Net estrogen effects on bone are probably a combination of direct and indirect effects on bone cells.

The mechanisms responsible for age-related bone loss are also multifactorial. Secondary hyperparathyroidism develops with aging because of decreased calcium absorption and vitamin D synthesis in elderly persons [7]. A recent multicenter study of postmenopausal women demonstrated that more than half of these subjects had vitamin D deficiency [14]. Aging is also associated with a decrease in stem cell precursors [15]. There seems to be a significant immune component with aging: the thymus atrophies and increased autoimmune destruction of bone tissue ensues [16].

Diagnosis

Multiple techniques have been used to assess fracture risk (Tables 1 and 2). Dual-energy X-ray absorptiometry (DEXA or DXA) is currently the most practical and cost-effective technique for bone density measurements. The technique involves the use of two x-ray beams of different energies. The attenuation of the x-ray beam passing through the bone compared with standards of known density permits estimation of the mineral

Table 1
Diagnosis of osteoporosis

Diagnostic technique	Advantages	Disadvantages
DXA	Standardized Widely available Low radiation exposure	Not a true volumetric measurement; density measurements are an estimate based on a two-dimensional projection
Quantitative CT	True volumetric measurements	Expensive Large radiation exposure
Peripheral quantitative CT	Less radiation exposure Less expensive Smaller	Can only measure peripheral skeleton density
Quantitative ultrasound • heel • tibia	No radiation Portable Easy and inexpensive for screening (health fairs)	Not standardized Lower sensitivity than DXA

Table 2
Clinical assessment tools for osteoporosis

Acronym	Stands for	Variables
OSIRIS	Osteoporosis index of risk	Age × –2 Weight (kg) × 2 (rounded down to nearest integer) Use of hormonal replacement therapy –2 History of fracture –2 If < –3 = high risk < +1 and > –3 = intermediate risk > +1 = low risk
OST	Osteoporosis self-assessment tool	Body weight (kg) Age (y) 0.2 × (body weight – age) <2 = high risk
SCORE	Simple calculated osteoporosis risk estimation	Race other than black: +5 Rheumatoid arthritis: +4 Nontraumatic fracture after age 45 years: +4 per fracture, up to a maximum of 12 Age: +3/decade Estrogen therapy: +1 if never Weight: –1 for each 4.5 kg >7 = high risk
ORAI	Osteoporosis risk assessment instrument	Age: ≥75 years: +15 65–74: +9 55–64: +5 Body weight: <60 kg: +9 60–70 kg: +3 ≥70: 0 Estrogen use: No = +2; yes = 0 >9 = high risk

content of the bone. The x-ray beam attenuation secondary to soft tissues surrounding the bone is subtracted from this measurement. The amount of radiation exposure is minimal; the effective dose has been calculated to be between 3.1 and 9.8 μSv depending on the site and scan mode [17]. By comparison, the radiation exposure from a chest radiograph is approximately 3.2×10^{-5} Sv. The DXA is useful for diagnosing osteoporosis and assessing fracture risk.

Bone density measurements are usually taken at the hip and spine. The World Health Organization developed criteria for the diagnosis of osteoporosis, which involved comparison of a patient's measured bone density to that of a young adult's peak reference values (T-score). The farther below this peak reference value (standard deviations) the patient is, the greater the fracture risk. A T-value of –1 or less is defined as normal; –2.5 or more is defined as osteoporosis; a T-score between –1 and –2.5 is in the gray zone or osteopenic range. Most DXA reports also include a Z-score, which is a comparison to a population of patients of the same age. The T-score is the best predictor of fracture risk; however, a Z-score should be used in patients younger than age 25. A Z-score more than –2 suggests that a secondary cause of osteoporosis is involved and that further diagnostic tests are warranted. Reference values for hip DXA measurements are based on the National Health and Nutrition Education Survey III database and are independent of DXA manufacturer.

DXA measurements have several significant weaknesses, including the fact that DXA is a two-dimensional image, and the measurements are not true volumetric measurements but rather an estimation. DXA measurements do not provide any structural information. Both of these DXA limitations are solved by the use of quantitative

CT measurements. These measurements have their own set of problems, however, including higher cost, higher radiation exposure, and greater time investment. Ironically, having a fragility fracture (spine, hip, wrists, forearms, shoulder, and ribs) is the single largest risk factor for development of a subsequent fracture. It is clear that better diagnostic techniques are necessary to identify patients who are at risk for fragility fractures.

Because patients who undergo dental procedures routinely have panoramic radiographs of the mandible, the use of this imaging technique to screen patients for osteoporosis has been investigated. It is estimated that approximately two thirds of the American population visit a dentist yearly and that many of these patients have dental radiographs as part of their examination [18]. If dental radiographs could be used as a screening tool for osteoporosis, they would be an invaluable tool for detecting patients at risk before they developed a fracture. Multiple indices have been proposed as being useful in identifying patients

who have osteoporosis (Table 3). Mandibular cortical thickness has been one of the more widely used measurements [19]. For this measurement a line is drawn from the midpoint of each mental foramen to the lower border of the mandible at right angles to the tangent to the lower border at this point [20]. The width of the cortical bone at the lower border is measured to the inner edge of the cortex. Devlin and Horner [21] found that the sensitivity and specificity of this technique in correctly identifying patients with low bone mass varied greatly depending on the values used as thresholds. If a mandibular cortical width (MCW) threshold of 3 mm or less was used, then the technique had a sensitivity of approximately 50% and a specificity of approximately 86%. In contrast, if an MCW of 4.5 mm was used, then the sensitivity of the technique was more than 95% but had a specificity of less than 20% [20]. This technique is hampered by the fact that there is significant interoperator variability. Attempts have been made to increase the sensitivity and specificity of MCW measurements by using an

Table 3
Assessment tools for dental panoramic radiographs

Measurement	Method	Features
Panoramic mandibular index, mental index, or MCW	A line is drawn from the midpoint of each mental foramen to the lower border of the mandible at right angles to the tangent to the lower border at this point. The width of the cortical bone at the lower border is measured to the inner edge of the cortex.	Most reliable of the mandibular cortical indices Sensitivity and specificity depend on MCW threshold used (3 vs 4.5 mm) Mental index shows a significant positive correlation with DXA measurements at spine and femur. However, not a substitute for DXA; could be useful for identifying patients who should have DXA
Gonial index or antegonial index	Thickness of the mandibular cortex at both angles of the mandible (gonial index) or more anteriorly in the antegonial region (antegonial index)	Antegonial index (but not gonial index) has been shown to have a significant positive correlation with bone mineral density measurements by DXA
Klemetti index	Appearance of the inferior mandibular cortex: **0**, normal, even, and sharp endosteal margin; **1**, moderately eroded, margin shows semilunar defects or seems to form endosteal cortical residues on one or both sides; **2**, severely eroded, the cortical layer forms heavy endosteal cortical residues and is clearly porous	Klemetti index of <2 is a good predictor of absence of osteoporosis on bone mineral density measurements (T score ≥1.5)

automated method to make the measurements because of the large interobserver variability [22]. Automated measurements seem to improve the reliability of these indices. A general limitation of these radiographic measurements is the relatively low sensitivity of this technique with changes in bone density in excess of 30% required for reliable discrimination [23].

Investigators also have tried to improve the sensitivity and specificity of radiographic techniques by combining them with various clinical risk indices, such as OSIRIS (osteoporosis index of risk), ORAI (osteoporosis risk assessment index), OST (osteoporosis self assessment tool), and SCORE (simple calculated osteoporosis risk estimation) (see Table 2). A recent European study reported on a 3-year trial that examined the power of the combination of OSIRIS plus MCW (OSTEODENT) in identifying patients with osteoporosis [20]. The OSTEODENT study found that although combining clinical and radiographic indices did improve specificity, sensitivity was negatively affected.

Taguchi and colleagues [24] also examined the correlation between dental radiographs and biochemical markers of bone turnover. These authors found a significant correlation between mandibular cortical erosion and width and spinal bone mineral density. There also was a positive correlation between mandibular cortical erosion and a biochemical marker for bone breakdown (urinary N-telopeptide cross-links of type I collagen) and bone formation (total alkaline phosphatase) [24].

Taken together, these data suggest that dental radiographs are a potentially useful way of screening for osteoporosis but that different practices must define for themselves—depending on their patient population—whether the emphasis should be placed on high sensitivity (and increased numbers of false-positive results) or high specificity (with increased numbers of false-negative results) in their screening and referral process. It is also likely that many patients being treated by dentists or oral surgeons are already on medication for osteoporosis. It is important for practitioners to be aware of potential dental implications of commonly used therapies.

Treatment of osteoporosis

Bone mass is determined by the net balance between bone formation, which is mediated by osteoblastic activity, and bone breakdown, which is mediated by osteoclastic activity. Current medications used to treat osteoporosis are generally grouped into two major categories: (1) those that inhibit osteoclastic activity (or antiresorptive agents) and (2) those that stimulate osteoblastic activity (anabolic agents). Most of the currently available agents to treat osteoporosis are antiresorptive agents. Only one anabolic agent, parathyroid hormone 1-34 (Forteo), is on the market in the United States. In my personal practice I generally use a stepped approach to therapy for osteoporosis. This suggested approach is only a general guideline and is not meant to be a rigid framework for treatment of osteoporosis. In Step 1, I make sure that all patients get adequate amounts of calcium, vitamin D, and exercise.

Recommended daily elemental calcium intake is between 1000 and 1300 mg, depending on age. The main source of dietary calcium is from dairy products (milk, 8 oz is approximately 300 mg; cheese, 1 oz is approximately 265 mg; yogurt, 6 oz is approximately 300 mg), although leafy green vegetables (collard greens, 1 cup is approximately 357 mg; turnip greens, 1 cup is approximately 249 mg; kale, 1 cup is approximately 179 mg) and nuts (almonds, 3 oz is approximately 210 mg) are additional sources of calcium. The two most common calcium supplements contain calcium carbonate (eg, Caltrate, OsCal, Tums) or calcium citrate (eg, Citracal). Calcium carbonate supplements are best split and taken two or three times per day with meals to improve absorption. Nutrients and minerals besides calcium are also important for bone health, so a balanced diet is essential.

Recommended vitamin D daily intake is 400 IU for patients between 51 and 70 years of age and 600 IU for patients older than 70 years of age [14]. It seems that larger doses of vitamin D are probably needed for optimal bone health, however, and an increase in the recommended daily dose of vitamin D to between 1000 and 2000 IU is currently under discussion. Recommended exercise regimens involve weight-bearing exercises (eg, walking, hiking, dancing) for at least 30 minutes 5 to 7 days per week. These measures by themselves increase bone mass by approximately 1% to 2% [25].

For Step 2 I use vitamin D analogs, selective estrogen receptor modulators, or estrogen (women) or testosterone (men). Multiple oral preparations of vitamin D are available, including cholecalciferol (D3), ergocalciferol (D2), calcitriol

(1,25 dihyroxyvitamin D), dihydrotachysterol, and doxecalciferol (Hectorol). In view of the high prevalence of vitamin D deficiency in the US population, it is worthwhile to screen postmenopausal patients for vitamin D levels [14]. In patients with vitamin D concentrations less than 20 ng/mL, I use ergocalciferol, 50,000 U, once per week for 8 weeks [26].

Selective estrogen receptor modulators are estrogen analogs that can serve either as agonists or antagonists of the estrogen receptor in a tissue-dependent manner. Tamoxifen was an early selective estrogen receptor modulator, although it is not currently indicated for the treatment of osteoporosis. Raloxifene has the beneficial effect of estrogens on bone without the side effects such as uterine bleeding or breast tenderness. Currently, raloxifene (Evista) and tamoxifen (Nolvadex, Valodex, Istubal) are the only US Food and Drug Administration–approved selective estrogen receptor modulators on the market, although others (eg, lasofoxifene) are currently under study. Raloxifene significantly decreases vertebral fracture risk and increases bone density between 1.35% and 2.5% [27].

Estrogens were the mainstay for the treatment of postmenopausal osteoporosis for many years and have been shown to be effective in fracture prevention. A National Institutes of Health–sponsored study, the Women's Health Initiative, demonstrated that although a conjugated estrogen/progesterone preparation (Prempro) decreased fracture risk, there was a moderate increase in the incidence of breast cancer, stroke, and heart attack [28]. Based on these findings, most professional societies do not currently recommend estrogen replacement therapy solely for fracture prevention, because other equally effective agents are available.

For Step 3 I use one of the bisphosphonates. Bisphosphonates are pyrophosphate analogs that interfere with protein prenylation and accelerate osteoclastic apoptosis [29]. Multiple oral and intravenous bisphosphonates are available. Oral bisphosphonates include once weekly preparations, such as alendronate (Fosamax) and risedronate (Actonel), and once monthly preparations, such as ibandronate (Boniva). Intravenous bisphosphonates include pamidronate (Aredia), zolendronate (Zometa), and ibandronate (Boniva). Pamidronate [29] and zoledronate [30] infusions have been shown to be effective in treating osteoporosis. Different infusion regimens have been tested, ranging from every 3 months to once per year. Data from the Horizon Pivotal Fracture Trial suggested that a 15-minute yearly infusion of 5 mg of zolendronate for osteoporosis is safe and effective for fracture prevention. Ibandronate is the only currently approved intravenous preparation for the treatment of postmenopausal osteoporosis, however, and it is given every 3 months [31]. Bisphosphonates can increase bone mineral density by 3% to 6%.

For Step 4 I use teriparatide or Forteo, which is synthetic parathyroid hormone (1-34). Teriparatide is the only currently available anabolic agent and is given as a daily subcutaneous injection (20 μg). Teriparatide increases bone mineral density at the spine, usually on the order of 9% to 13% [32].

These therapeutic options do not necessarily need to be followed in a sequential manner. Many factors determine which medication a patient receives initially, including severity of osteoporosis, history of fractures, and risk factors, such as family history of breast cancer. In these latter patients, Evista has been shown to be as effective as tamoxifen in chemoprevention for invasive breast cancer [33]. Some of these medications also can be used in combination, such as vitamin D and bisphosphonates or raloxifene and teriparatide [34]. Some combinations, such as teriparatide and bisphosphonates, actually seem to antagonize each other's beneficial effect on bone mass, however [35]. Treatment of patients who have osteoporosis requires a thorough initial evaluation and follow-up.

Impact of therapy for osteoporosis on oral health

Multiple medications are used to treat osteoporosis, and many of these medications may have a direct effect on dental health. Because of space limitations, this discussion focuses on three commonly used osteoporosis treatments: (1) estrogens, (2) bisphosphonates, and (3) teriparatide.

For many years estrogens were the mainstay of treatment of postmenopausal patients with osteoporosis. A study by Paganini-Hill [36] examined the impact of estrogen replacement on the teeth of postmenopausal women and found that patients on estrogen had a significantly lower risk of having fewer than 25 teeth (RR 0.76). A prospective study by Grodstein and colleagues [37] in postmenopausal women also found that estrogen was protective against tooth loss (RR 0.73 for hormone replacement therapy users versus nonusers). Another prospective study by

Lopez-Marcos and colleagues [38] examined the effects of hormone replacement therapy (as a patch) on 210 female menopausal patients (aged 40–58) with periodontal disease. The authors found that although hormone replacement therapy did not improve gingival recession, it was protective against increased tooth mobility. Estrogen does not seem to have a negative impact on dental health and may be of benefit in certain conditions.

Although bisphosphonates are clearly beneficial for treating osteoporosis, they are currently the medication of most concern because of their potential impact on dental health. The potent nitrogen-containing bisphosphonates are pyrophosphate analogs that induce osteoclastic apoptosis by inhibiting the enzyme farnesyl diphosphate synthase (FPP synthase) and decrease the levels of geranylgeranyl diphosphate, which is required for GTPase prenylation and subsequent translocation to the cell membrane [39]. Periodontitis is an inflammatory process characterized by loss of the attachment of the tooth to the alveolar bone and bone loss. Because osteoclasts are activated by the inflammatory process in the gingiva and are responsible for dental bone resorption, it has been proposed that bisphosphonates might be useful in periodontitis to prevent this bone loss. In the few trials that have been performed it seems that bisphosphonates are useful in the management of periodontitis [40,41].

Recent reports have highlighted a serious bisphosphonate-induced side effect, however, which has been termed osteonecrosis of the jaw. It is still a relatively poorly defined condition characterized by necrosis of the bone in the maxilla, mandible, or both and seems to be precipitated by loss of vascular supply to the affected bone. Patients usually present with pain and bleeding [42], and the mandible is more commonly involved than the maxilla [43]. Many of these patients have history of cancer (in particular, multiple myeloma or metastatic breast or prostate cancer) or have received radiotherapy or chemotherapy [44]. It has also been reported to occur more frequently in patients undergoing dental procedures. Osteonecrosis of the jaw has been reported to occur in patients without any of these risk factors except the use of bisphosphonates, however. Men and women can be affected [45]. The more potent nitrogen-containing bisphosphonates seem to be more closely associated with this condition (94% of cases [43]) and include zolendronate, pamidronate, and alendronate [44].

Factors predisposing to bisphosphonate-induced osteonecrosis of the jaw are duration of therapy (may have cumulative effects), intravenous preparation (higher delivered dose), and dental procedures (60% of cases) [43].

Management should be conservative with antibiotics and limited débridement [46]. Patients with malignancy or osteoporosis who are about to start bisphosphonate therapy should have a baseline dental examination, and any dental procedures preferably should be completed before initiation of the bisphosphonate [47]. For patients already on bisphosphonates, no evidence suggests that stopping the medication before a dental procedure is of benefit, especially when one takes into account the long half-life of this medication in bone. Currently there are insufficient data to indicate how significant a problem this is.

Teriparatide is a potent anabolic agent for the treatment of osteoporosis. Animal data also suggest that parathyroid hormone may be of benefit in accelerating fracture healing [48]. Studies in rats suggest that parathyroid hormone increases alveolar bone mass and prevents bone loss after a dental extraction [49]. Parathyroid hormone also has been shown to be effective in preventing dental bone loss associated with periodontitis [50,51]. There are no current prospective studies in human subjects, but experimental data support a role for parathyroid hormone as a promising anabolic agent for the prevention of alveolar bone loss.

Role of the oral surgeon in the diagnosis and management of patients with osteoporosis

The state of health of the oral cavity is frequently a reflection of patients' general health and can give important clues to many systemic diseases. Periodontal disease has been associated with cardiovascular disease, diabetes mellitus, poor pregnancy outcomes, and osteoporosis [52]. Multiple studies have examined whether there is a correlation between osteoporosis and tooth loss. Presumably the same systemic factors that lead to bone loss in the skeleton also would result in bone loss in the teeth. The mandibular bone has a greater cortical thickness than the maxillary bone, and bone loss is detected earlier in the latter bone [23]. A study by Krall and colleagues [53] examined whether there was any correlation between bone density and tooth loss in 329 postmenopausal women. These authors found a significant positive correlation between spinal and radial bone mineral density and the number of remaining teeth. This study also reported that although there was no significant correlation between bone mineral density and use of dentures in the study population as a whole, patients who required dentures after the age of 40 had significantly lower spinal bone mineral density [53]. These same authors also reported that for each 1% drop in bone mineral density in the whole body, femoral neck, or spine, the relative risk of losing a tooth increased by 4.83, 1.50, or 1.45, respectively [54]. These data suggest that patients who have osteoporosis are at a higher risk of developing tooth problems.

A related question is whether patients who have osteoporosis and are undergoing a dental procedure are at higher risk of poor healing or complications. For example, do osteoporotic patients who have dental implants have impaired osseointegration? This is a controversial area, and conflicting results have been reported. Available data suggest that osteoporotic patients heal normally [55]. It is likely, however, that the most important factor for determining healing and osseointegration potential relates to the underlying cause of osteoporosis (eg, glucocorticoid, estrogen deficiency) rather than the mere presence of osteoporosis.

In summary, dental bone loss correlates with systemic bone loss. Oral surgeons can play an important role in the screening and diagnosis of these patients with osteoporosis. In view of recent awareness of osteonecrosis of the jaw as a side effect of bisphosphonates used to treat patients who have osteoporosis, it is important for oral surgeons to team up with medical practitioners who are following the patients. It is important for physicians to evaluate osteoporotic patients for dental procedures before initiation of therapy and oral surgeons to develop a treatment plan with physicians to co-manage patients already on a bisphosphonate before extensive oral surgery.

References

[1] Administration on Aging, US Department of Health and Human Services. A profile of older Americans: Available at: http://www.aoa.gov/prof/Statistics/statistics.asp.

[2] Hui SL, Slemenda CW, Johnston CC Jr. Age and bone mass as predictors of fracture in a prospective study. J Clin Invest 1988;81:1804–9.

[3] Kanis JA and the WHO Study Group. Assessment of fracture risk and its application to screening for postmenopausal osteoporosis: report of a WHO Study Group. World Health Organ Tech Rep Ser 1994;843:1–129.

[4] Ross PD, Davis JW, Epstein RS, et al. Pre-existing fractures and bone mass predict vertebral fracture incidence in women. Ann Intern Med 1991;114:919–23.

[5] Lindsay R, Silverman SL, Cooper C, et al. Risk of new vertebral fracture in the year following a fracture. JAMA 2001;285:320–3.

[6] NIH Consensus Development Panel. Osteoporosis prevention, diagnosis, and therapy. JAMA 2001; 285:785–95.

[7] Riggs BL, Khosla S, Melton LJ 3rd. Sex steroids and the construction and conservation of the adult skeleton. Endocr Rev 2002;23:279–302.

[8] Recker R, Lappe J, Davies K, et al. Characterization of perimenopausal bone loss: a prospective study. J Bone Miner Res 2000;15:1965–73.

[9] Blair HC, Robinson LJ, Zaidi M. Osteoclast signalling pathways. Biochem Biophys Res Commun 2005;328:728–38.

[10] Raisz LG. Pathogenesis of osteoporosis: concepts, conflicts, and prospects. J Clin Invest 2005;115: 3318–25.

[11] Zallone A. Direct and indirect estrogen actions on osteoblasts and osteoclasts. Ann N Y Acad Sci 2006;1068:173–9.

[12] Weitzmann MN, Pacifici R. Estrogen regulation of immune cell bone interactions. Ann N Y Acad Sci 2006;1068:256–74.

[13] Weitzmann MN, Pacifici R. Estrogen deficiency and bone loss: an inflammatory tale. J Clin Invest 2006; 116:1186–94.

[14] Holick MF, Siris ES, Binkley N, et al. Prevalence of vitamin D inadequacy among postmenopausal North American women receiving osteoporosis therapy. J Clin Endocrinol Metab 2005;90:3215–24.

[15] Blair HC, Carrington JL. Bone cell precursors and the pathophysiology of bone loss. Ann N Y Acad Sci 2006;1068:244–9.

[16] Clowes JA, Riggs BL, Khosla S. The role of the immune system in the pathophysiology of osteoporosis. Immunol Rev 2005;208:207–27.

[17] Blake GM, Naeem M, Boutros M. Comparison of effective dose to children and adults from dual X-ray absorptiometry examinations. Bone 2006;38:935–42.

[18] White SC, Taguchi A, Kao D, et al. Clinical and panoramic predictors of femur bone mineral density. Osteoporos Int 2005;16:339–46.

[19] Klemetti E, Kolmakov S, Kroger H. Pantomography in assessment of the osteoporosis risk group. Scand J Dent Res 1994;102:68–72.

[20] Karayianni K, Horner K, Mitsea A, et al. Accuracy in osteoporosis diagnosis of a combination of mandibular cortical width measurement on dental panoramic radiographs and a clinical risk index (OSIRIS): the OSTEODENT project. Bone 2007;40:223–9.

[21] Devlin H, Horner K. Mandibular radiomorphometric indices in the diagnosis of reduced skeletal bone mineral density. Osteoporos Int 2002;13:373–8.

[22] Devlin H, Allen PD, Graham J, et al. Automated osteoporosis risk assessment by dentists: a new pathway to diagnosis. Bone 2007;40:835–42.

[23] Bodic F, Hamel L, Lerouxel E, et al. Bone loss and teeth. Joint Bone Spine 2005;72:215–21.

[24] Taguchi A, Sanada M, Krall E, et al. Relationship between dental panoramic radiographic findings and biochemical markers of bone turnover. J Bone Miner Res 2003;18:1689–94.

[25] Shea B, Wells G, Cranney A, et al. Meta-analyses of therapies for postmenopausal osteoporosis. VII. Meta-analysis of calcium supplementation for the prevention of postmenopausal osteoporosis. Endocr Rev 2002;23:552–9.

[26] Malabanan A, Veronikis IE, Holick MF. Redefining vitamin D insufficiency. Lancet 1998;351:805–6.

[27] Cranney A, Tugwell P, Zytaruk N, et al. Meta-analyses of therapies for postmenopausal osteoporosis. IV. Meta-analysis of raloxifene for the prevention and treatment of postmenopausal osteoporosis. Endocr Rev 2002;23:524–8.

[28] Anderson GL, Limacher M, Assaf AR, et al. Effects of conjugated equine estrogen in postmenopausal women with hysterectomy: the Women's Health Initiative randomized controlled trial. JAMA 2004;291: 1701–12.

[29] Rogers MJ, Frith JC, Luckman SP, et al. Molecular mechanisms of action of bisphosphonates. Bone 1999;24:73S–9S.

[30] Saag K, Lindsay R, Kriegman A, et al. A single zoledronic acid infusion reduces bone resorption markers more rapidly than weekly oral alendronate in postmenopausal women with low bone mineral density. Bone 2007;40:1238–43.

[31] Adami S, Felsenberg D, Christiansen C, et al. Efficacy and safety of ibandronate given by intravenous injection once every 3 months. Bone 2004;34:881–9.

[32] Neer RM, Arnaud CD, Zanchetta JR, et al. Effect of parathyroid hormone (1-34) on fractures and bone mineral density in postmenopausal women with osteoporosis. N Engl J Med 2001;344:1434–41.

[33] Vogel VG, Costantino JP, Wickerham DL, et al. Effects of tamoxifen vs raloxifene on the risk of developing invasive breast cancer and other disease outcomes: the NSABP Study of Tamoxifen and Raloxifene (STAR) P-2 trial. JAMA 2006;295: 2727–41.

[34] Deal C, Omizo M, Schwartz EN, et al. Combination teriparatide and raloxifene therapy for postmenopausal osteoporosis: results from a 6-month double-blind placebo-controlled trial. J Bone Miner Res 2005;20:1905–11.

[35] Finkelstein JS, Hayes A, Hunzelman JL, et al. The effects of parathyroid hormone, alendronate, or both in men with osteoporosis. N Engl J Med 2003;349:1216–26.

[36] Paganini-Hill A. The benefits of estrogen replacement therapy on oral health: the Leisure World cohort. Arch Intern Med 1995;155:2325–9.

[37] Grodstein F, Colditz GA, Stampfer MJ. Post-menopausal hormone use and tooth loss: a prospective study. J Am Dent Assoc 1996;127:370–7, quiz 92.

[38] Lopez-Marcos JF, Garcia-Valle S, Garcia-Iglesias AA. Periodontal aspects in menopausal women undergoing hormone replacement therapy. Med Oral Patol Oral Cir Bucal 2005;10:132–41.

[39] Coxon FP, Thompson K, Rogers MJ. Recent advances in understanding the mechanism of action of bisphosphonates. Curr Opin Pharmacol 2006;6:307–12.

[40] Lane N, Armitage GC, Loomer P, et al. Bisphosphonate therapy improves the outcome of conventional periodontal treatment: results of a 12-month, randomized, placebo-controlled study. J Periodontol 2005;76:1113–22.

[41] Reddy MS, Geurs NC, Gunsolley JC. Periodontal host modulation with antiproteinase, anti-inflammatory, and bone-sparing agents: a systematic review. Ann Periodontol 2003;8:12–37.

[42] Merigo E, Manfredi M, Meleti M, et al. Jaw bone necrosis without previous dental extractions associated with the use of bisphosphonates (pamidronate and zoledronate): a four-case report. J Oral Pathol Med 2005;34:613–7.

[43] Woo SB, Hellstein JW, Kalmar JR. Narrative review: bisphosphonates and osteonecrosis of the jaws. Ann Intern Med 2006;144:753–61.

[44] Marx RE, Sawatari Y, Fortin M, et al. Bisphosphonate-induced exposed bone (osteonecrosis/osteopetrosis) of the jaws: risk factors, recognition, prevention, and treatment. J Oral Maxillofac Surg 2005;63:1567–75.

[45] Merigo E, Manfredi M, Meleti M, et al. Bone necrosis of the jaws associated with bisphosphonate treatment: a report of twenty-nine cases. Acta Biomed 2006;77:109–17.

[46] Dunstan CR, Felsenberg D, Seibel MJ. Therapy insight: the risks and benefits of bisphosphonates for the treatment of tumor-induced bone disease. Nat Clin Pract Oncol 2007;4:42–55.

[47] Migliorati CA, Casiglia J, Epstein J, et al. Managing the care of patients with bisphosphonate-associated osteonecrosis: an American Academy of Oral Medicine position paper. J Am Dent Assoc 2005;136: 1658–68.

[48] Alkhiary YM, Gerstenfeld LC, Krall E, et al. Enhancement of experimental fracture-healing by systemic administration of recombinant human parathyroid hormone (PTH 1-34). J Bone Joint Surg Am 2005;87:731–41.

[49] Kawane T, Takahashi S, Saitoh H, et al. Anabolic effects of recombinant human parathyroid hormone (1-84) and synthetic human parathyroid hormone (1-34) on the mandibles of osteopenic ovariectomized rats with maxillary molar extraction. Horm Metab Res 2002;34:293–302.

[50] Barros SP, Silva MA, Somerman MJ, et al. Parathyroid hormone protects against periodontitis-associated bone loss. J Dent Res 2003;82:791–5.

[51] Marques MR, da Silva MA, Manzi FR, et al. Effect of intermittent PTH administration in the periodontitis-associated bone loss in ovariectomized rats. Arch Oral Biol 2005;50:421–9.

[52] Kim J, Amar S. Periodontal disease and systemic conditions: a bidirectional relationship. Odontology 2006;94:10–21.

[53] Krall EA, Dawson-Hughes B, Papas A, et al. Tooth loss and skeletal bone density in healthy postmenopausal women. Osteoporos Int 1994;4:104–9.

[54] Krall EA, Garcia RI, Dawson-Hughes B. Increased risk of tooth loss is related to bone loss at the whole body, hip, and spine. Calcif Tissue Int 1996;59: 433–7.

[55] Mombelli A, Cionca N. Systemic diseases affecting osseointegration therapy. Clin Oral Implants Res 2006;17(Suppl 2):97–103.

ELSEVIER
SAUNDERS

Oral Maxillofacial Surg Clin N Am 19 (2007) 487–498

ORAL AND
MAXILLOFACIAL
SURGERY CLINICS
of North America

Bisphosphonates and Bisphosphonate Induced Osteonecrosis

Yoh Sawatari, DDS*, Robert E. Marx, DDS

Division of Oral and Maxillofacial Surgery, University of Miller Miami School of Medicine, Deering Medical Plaza, 9380 SW 150th Street, Suite 190, Miami, FL 33157, USA

Bisphosphonates are extensively used in medicine via two routes. The intravenous amino-bisphosphonates pamidronate (Aredia) and zoledronate (Zometa) are cleared by the US Food and Drug Administration (FDA) to contain the proliferation of metastatic cancer deposits in bone and reduce the hypercalcemia of malignancy [1,2]. The more common malignances in which these drugs are used are multiple myeloma and metastatic breast cancer, but they are also sometimes used for metastatic prostate, lung, and kidney cancers. They occasionally have been used "off label" (used for an indication not cleared by the FDA) to theoretically prevent metastasis to bone and treat osteopenia or osteoporosis in patients who do not have cancer [3].

The oral aminobisphosphonates alendronate (Fosamax), residronate (Actonel), and ibandronate (Boniva) are cleared by the FDA for the treatment of osteopenia/osteoporosis. Some also have been used "off label" to treat cancer deposits in bone and Paget's disease of bone and have been suggested to treat periodontal bone loss [4]. The specific oral bisphosphonates etidronate (Didronel) and tiludronate (Skelid) are cleared by the FDA only for control of Paget's disease in bone and to treat heterotopic bone formations. They are not aminobisphosphonates because they do not contain nitrogen in their side chain and are less potent. These two bisphosphonates have not been shown to produce osteonecrosis of the jaw.

The intravenous aminobisphosphonates anti-resorptive action, which prevents pathologic bone resorption, has improved quality of life significantly and even extended the life of many cancer patients [5]. This same antiresorptive effect, which is mediated through the toxic death of normal osteoclasts, also prevents normal bone remodeling and renewal, however, which results in osteonecrosis in the target areas of the jaw [6]. Similarly, the oral aminobisphosphonates have significantly reduced fracture incidence and the pain and disability in women with osteoporosis [7]. Because oral aminobisphosphonates are also toxic to osteoclasts, they have created many cases of bisphosphonate-induced osteonecrosis of the jaws (BIONJ) [8].

Bisphosphonate-induced osteonecrosis by the dates and numbers

The first reports of osteonecrosis of the jaws caused by bisphosphonates were by Marx in September 2003 (Fig. 1) [9]. Although this finding was initially met with some skepticism, particularly by some of the drug manufacturers [10], confirming articles from across the world [11,12] were underscored by three separate publications that appeared in the December 2004 issue of the *Journal of the American Dental Association* [13–15]. As of May 2007, more than 300 publications linked bisphosphonates to osteonecrosis in the jaws, and an estimated 10,000 individual cases were reported. Most specialties of dentistry had posted definitions or position papers, as did three medical organizations, including the Mayo Clinic, the American Society for Bone and

_____

* Corresponding author.

E-mail address: ysawatari@med.miami.edu
(Y. Sawatari).

1042-3699/07/$ - see front matter © 2007 Elsevier Inc. All rights reserved.
doi:10.1016/j.coms.2007.07.003

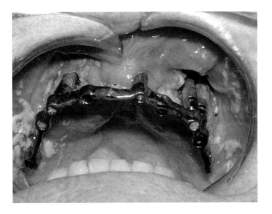

Fig. 1. Exposed necrotic bone caused by zoledronate (Zometa) therapy for multiple myeloma.

Mineral Research, and the American Society of Endocrinology.

The true incidence of bisphosphonate-induced osteonecrosis is not known and will likely never be known accurately because the number of patients receiving these drugs is not recorded. Many cases of osteonecrosis are not reported. The original drug performance data advanced to the FDA from the drug companies' studies did not include an oral examination or any report forms that listed osteonecrosis as a possibility. Publications have estimated a wide incidence range for intravenous bisphosphonate-induced osteonecrosis from as little as 0.8% [16] to as much as 30% [17]; for oral aminobisphosphonate-induced osteonecrosis the incidence has been reported to be between 0.007% and 0.01% [18]. The median between these wide ranges is most likely to be closer to being accurate with an incidence for intravenous bisphosphonates at 8% and for oral bisphosphonates at 0.015%. These relatively low incidence estimates are balanced against the large numbers of patients who currently receive bisphosphonates. Sales records estimate that 3 million individuals have received or are receiving intravenous bisphosphonates worldwide and that 13 million women in the United States alone (and many millions more in Europe) are currently receiving bisphosphonates.

The mechanism of bisphosphonate-induced osteonecrosis

The mechanism of bisphosphonate toxicity to bone common to oral and intravenous aminobisphosphonates is death of osteoclasts [19,20]. This drug effect is the same one that provides their therapeutic effects. Cancer proliferation in bone is caused by the cancer's elaboration of receptor activator nuclear Kappa-b ligand (RANKL), which normally activates the receptor activator nuclear Kappa-b (RANK) receptors on the osteoclast cell membrane to actively resorb bone and create resorption cavities into which the cancer proliferates (Fig. 2) [18]. If an accumulation of bisphosphonates is absorbed into the bone matrix surface, however, osteoclasts ingest it at the start of bone resorption and rapidly succumb, which prevents any resorption. In osteoporosis, the bisphosphonates also inhibit osteoclast-mediated bone resorption, which reduces the gradual reduction in bone mass with ageing and menopause in women. This results in a more mineralized and somewhat stronger bone initially but also can result in the accumulation of older, more brittle bone over many years.

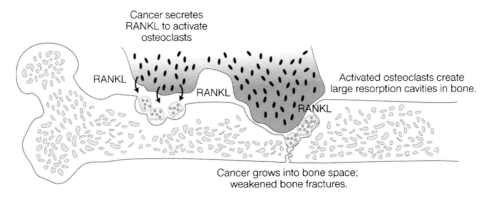

Fig. 2. The mechanism and cancer resorption in bone is often mediated through stimulation of normal osteoclasts by the secretion of RANKL by the cancer.

The toxic effect on osteoclasts is mostly on mature osteoclasts as they resorb bone but also extends to osteoclast precursors in the bone marrow [20]. This toxicity is caused by interruption of the Mevalonate branch pathway, which is vital to the survival of osteoclasts because it produces isoprenoid lipids [20,21]. The specific point in this pathway is primarily the inhibition of the farnesyl synthetase enzyme, which after several downstream synthetic steps results in geranyl-geranyl proteins, which comprise part of the isoprenoid lipids [20].

Pertinent chemistry of bisphosphonates

The molecular structure of bisphosphonates is a simple one that explains its absorption, distribution, and clinical findings related to osteonecrosis. Bisphosphonates are related to pyrophosphates, which are diphosphonates such as technetium-99 methylene diphosphonate commonly used in bone scans because of their uptake in active bone turnover. Pyrophosphates are rapidly hydrolyzed in the body. Substituting a carbon atom for the oxygen atom in the backbone of the pyrophosphate molecule turns it into a bisphosphonate, however, and makes hydrolysis impossible (Fig. 3). Bisphosphonates are not metabolized in the body at all, yet they retain their affinity for bone. The carbon atom

further adds to bisphosphonate bone affinity by binding to hydroxyapatite crystals in bone, which is further enhanced to an irreversible binding if a hydroxyl group (OH) is added to the carbon's R-1 position (Fig. 4) [18,22]. This result is the case in all bisphosphonates that have produced BIONJ to date. Bisphosphonates are rapidly bound to bone and can be removed only by acid dissolution, of which only osteoclasts have the capability. The toxicity of bisphosphonates is selective for osteoclasts. The R-2 position on this backbone carbon atom relates to potency [22,23]. Nitrogen atoms in the side chain in this position increase potency. The two non–nitrogen-containing bisphosphonates etidronate (Didronel) and tiludronate (Skelid) are the least potent. Studies that determined Didronel to be the least potent also determined the oral bisphosphonate Fosamax (most commonly known to produce BIONJ) to be 5000 times more potent and Zometa (an intravenous bisphosphonate most commonly known to produce BIONJ) to be 10,000 times more potent.

Clinical disease and onset of bisphosphonate-induced osteonecrosis of the jaws

Clinical disease is exposed bone that fails to heal despite local care with or without antibiotics. The working definition of BIONJ put forth the by

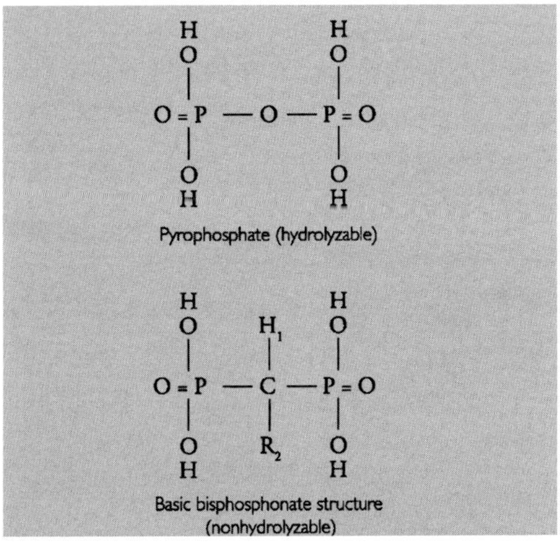

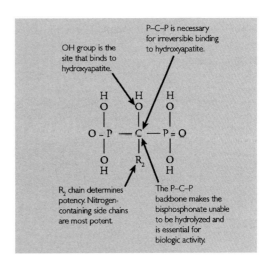

Fig. 3. The substitution of a carbon atom in the backbone of the pyrophosphate molecule makes it nonhydrolyzable and a true bisphosphonate.

Fig. 4. The basic bisphosphonate molecule. An OH onto the R-1 position of the backbone carbon increases its affinity for bone, and side chains with nitrogen on the R2 position add potency.

the American Association of Oral and Maxillofacial Surgeons is "exposed bone in the maxilla or mandible that fails to heal within eight weeks in a patient receiving or who has received a systemic bisphosphonate and who has not received local radiation therapy to the jaws" [23]. An intravenous dose of 90 mg of Aredia provided monthly and 4 mg of Zometa provided monthly are considered equal potent doses. It takes approximately six monthly doses of intravenous bisphosphonates to place a patient at risk for BIONJ [24], which is contrasted to the 3 years or 156 continuous weekly doses that are required to place patients who take Fosamax or Actonel into the risk range for BIONJ [8,18]. This difference is caused by the low lipid solubility of oral bisphosphonates, which limits their absorption in the small intestines to only 0.63%. Oral bisphosphonates accumulate in the bone much more slowly, and clinically exposed bone does not appear until after a 3-year exposure, with the incidence and severity increasing with each additional year of drug use [8,18].

Bisphosphonate-induced osteonecrosis always begins in the alveolar bone, where it may extend to the inferior border or rami of the mandible or into the zygoma or maxillary sinus walls about the maxilla (Fig. 5). This development is caused by the greater bone turnover rate and greater reliance on osteoclast-mediated remodeling in the alveolar bone, which results from the pressure and tension forces placed on the alveolar bone by occlusion or denture wearing [25,26]. The remodeling rate of alveolar bone in animal models has been shown to be ten times that of long bones, such as the tibia [27]. Hyperocclusion, periodontal inflammation, failing root canal fills, abscesses, and surgical trauma—all of which increase the rate of bone turnover in alveolar bone [25,26,28]—are also known to initiate events in the development of BIONJ. Early radiographic signs of a widened periodontal ligament space and sclerosis of the lamina dura attest to alveolar bone as the starting point of BIONJ (Fig. 6). Early clinical signs of deep bone pain about teeth or tooth mobility unexplained by dental or other pathologies are also early indications of bisphosphonate toxicity.

Bisphosphonate-induced osteonecrosis occurs more frequently in mandibular than maxillary sites by a ratio of 2:1 [24]. The exposed bone may be extensive or relatively small, with some cases subtly presenting with only a pinpoint exposure that belies a greater amount of necrotic bone beneath. Although pain is more likely with greater amounts of exposed bone, the exposed bone by itself is necrotic, deinnervated bone that is not painful but becomes painful when colonized by micro-organisms or when an actual infection develops. The most frequent micro-organisms found on the exposed bone are *Actinomyces*, *Viellonella*, *Eikenella*, and *Moraxella* species, all of which are most sensitive to penicillin (Fig. 7). This finding has been the basis of much of the nonsurgical management of BIONJ.

Incorrect and confusing terms

Unfortunately, newly discovered diseases are often given names and acronyms by associations and interest groups before they understand the pathophysiology. Many readers remember the terms *AIDS-related complex* (ARC) and *human T-cell lymphotropic virus-related disease* (HILV-RD), which are currently known as HIV

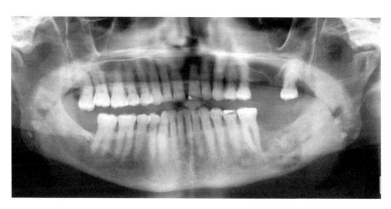

Fig. 5. This panoramic film shows the pattern of BIONJ appearing first and more extensively in the alveolar bone then extending to the inferior border.

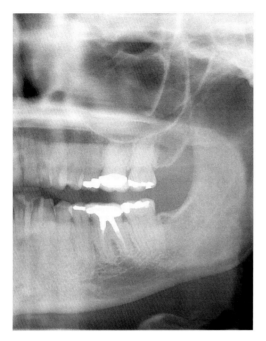

Fig. 6. Sclerosis of the lamina dura and widening of the periodontal membrane space are seen in this patient taking a bisphosphonate.

infection or actual AIDS. Such has been the case with BIONJ.

Such incorrect terminology already has created uncertainty and confusion as to the cause and diagnosis of this drug complication and requires clarification. Several organizations and publications have advanced the term "bisphosphonate-related osteonecrosis of the jaws" [23]. This term is incorrect because low hemoglobin may be

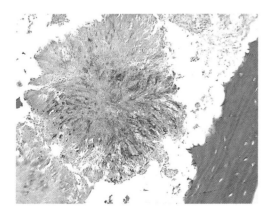

Fig. 7. Colony of Actinomyces organisms seen on the surface of the necrotic bone in a BIONJ case.

related to anemia but does not cause it, and low bone mass is related to osteoporosis but is not the cause—but rather the result—of the osteoporosis. Similarly, terms such as "bisphosphonate-associated osteonecrosis" [13], "osteochemonecrosis" [29], and "avascular bone necrosis" [12] also have been advanced. Bisphosphonate-associated osteonecrosis is incorrect because impacted teeth are associated with cleidocranial dysplasia but they do not cause it. Similarly, pain is associated with abscessed teeth but the pain does not cause the abscess. Osteochemonecrosis is not a precise term either because the bisphosphonate is not directly caustic or toxic to the bone. Its toxicity is directed at osteoclasts, in which its lost contribution to bone renewal produces the osteonecrosis. This term also implies a causal role for chemotherapy, which is not the case. Finally, the term "avascular bone necrosis" is incorrect, because although the dead bone is absent of blood vessels, the loss of blood vessels is not the cause of the bone death. Instead, bone death is caused by absent osteoclast function, which in turn is the cause of the blood vessel loss. BIONJ is the only correct term and the preferred term because it indicates the true cause-and-effect relationship between certain bisphosphonates and osteonecrosis of the jaws.

Prevention and treatment of intravenous bisphosphonate-induced osteonecrosis

The osteonecrosis induced by intravenous bisphosphonates is generally more extensive, more severe, more unresponsive to discontinuation of the drug, and less responsive to surgical débridement. These characteristics are likely caused by the intravenous route, which allows a 40% bioavailability compared with the oral route, which allows a 0.63% bioavailability (a 64-fold increase in bioavailability). Concentrations accumulate in bone much more rapidly and the ability of the bone marrow to replace dead osteoclasts becomes exhausted, with time rendering the osteonecrosis irreversible even if the drug is discontinued.

Prevention and treatment guidelines already have been published and are based on the data concerning dental comorbidities and the initiating event that resulted in the exposed bone [8,18,24]. Approximately 25% of BIONJ cases develop spontaneously, whereas 75% of cases are initiated by a dental pathologic condition or surgical procedure [25], including tooth extractions,

Table 1
Initiating event

1. Spontaneous	30/119 (25.2%)
2. Tooth removal	45/119 (37.8%)
3. Active periodontitis	34/119 (28.6%)
4. Periodontal surgery	5/119 (11.2%)
5. Dental implant	4/119 (3.4%)
6. Apicoectomy	1/119 (0.8%)

periodontal surgery, untreated periodontal inflammation, abscessed teeth, failed root canal fills, and apical surgery (Table 1). Control of these pathologic conditions so as to arrest them before bisphosphonate therapy and prevent the need for oral surgical procedures during bisphosphonate therapy helps prevent up to 75% of cases.

Prevention recommendations before intravenous bisphosphonate therapy

Because metastatic deposits in bone are often recognized early and proliferate somewhat slowly, and because four to six monthly doses of intravenous bisphosphonate are required to significantly affect bone healing in the jaws, there is sufficient time for dentists and dental specialists to prepare the oral cavity. It is recommended that dental professionals and medical oncologists open more regular lines of communication and that medical oncologists refer such patients to qualified dentists for care during this early stage of therapy. Dentists should develop a treatment plan focused on correcting pathologic conditions and stabilizing the dentition to prevent the need for invasive procedures after 4 to 6 months of bisphosphonate therapy. Teeth that are nonrestorable, abscessed, have failing root canal fills, or are periodontally unsalvageable should be removed as a first priority. Next should follow periodontal care to arrest periodontal inflammation, salvage treatable teeth, and educate patients regarding self-maintenance. Restorative and prosthodontic procedures can follow and be accomplished well into intravenous bisphosphonate therapy. New dental implant placements and adult orthodontics pose a significant risk in this patient population and are not recommended, however.

Prevention recommendation during intravenous bisphosphonate therapy

Once a patient has received four to six doses of an intravenous bisphosphonate, there is significant suppression of bone turnover in the alveolar bone, which makes bone healing unpredictable and risky for osteonecrosis. During this phase of intravenous bisphosphonate therapy, avoiding invasive oral surgical procedures, including tooth extractions, dental implant placements, periodontal surgery, ridge augmentation grafts, and apical surgeries, which have been known to initiate BIONJ in these patients [24], is recommended unless there is no alternative. Because restorative procedures such as crowns, bridges, and removable partial and full dentures do not involve invasive procedures, they pose no direct risk and are actually recommended to prevent the need for future surgical procedures. Adult orthodontic procedures are not recommended in these patients.

Teeth that are nonrestorable are better treated with a root canal fill and crown amputation than with extraction. Similarly, teeth with mobility are best splinted—if practical—rather than extracted, and failing root canal fills should be reinstrumented and refilled as opposed to extracted or treated by apical surgery. If extraction is unavoidable, patients should be informed of the risks of BIONJ and a consent form should be signed.

Treatment of established intravenous bisphosphonate-induced osteonecrosis of the jaws

Because 25% of BIONJ cases develop without an initiating event and many patients do not gain access to preventive measures, treating BIONJ is inevitable for most practitioners. The goal of treatment is to prevent or alleviate pain, reduce infections, and stabilize the progression of exposed bone (Fig. 8). This treatment begins

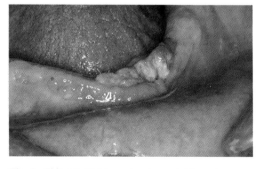

Fig. 8. This exposed bone has been stable and asymptomatic for 3 years with 0.12% chlorhexidine mouth rinses and penicillin V-K antibiotic courses despite continued Zometa therapy.

with informing patients that the intravenous bisphosphonate has been beneficial to them by containing their metastatic cancer despite the osteonecrosis for which they require treatment. They should be informed that they may need several dental specialists to maintain the rest of their oral health and they must begin a self-maintenance schedule to reduce the possibility of second or third sites developing. Patients must expect frequent follow-up visits (approximately every 4 months) and must comply with medications. We also inform patients that exposed bone is likely to be permanent and requires ongoing monitoring and medications for control; in some cases, a bony resection may be necessary.

Because the exposed bone is not painful unless heavily colonized or infected, patients who present without pain are treated with only a 0.12% chlorhexidine (Peridex) 30-mL swish-and-spit regimen three times daily. If pain and infection are present, penicillin VK, 500 mg, four times daily is added to the 0.12% chlorhexidine regimen. This formulation of penicillin is non-toxic and is compatible with long-term usage (years) without "super infections" or the development of candidiasis. It may be used ongoing in severe cases. As an alternative or if a patient is concerned about long-term antibiotic use, it may be used only during episodes of pain. If a patient is penicillin allergic, our experience has shown that levoflaxacin (Levaquin), 500 mg, once daily is the best alternative. Other reasonably effective alternatives are doxycycline (Vibramycin), 100 mg, daily or zithromycin (Zithromax), 250 mg, daily. Use of levaquin or zithromax should be limited to a course of 21 days or less because of the potential for liver enzyme elevations, however. Clindamycin is not recommended because of absent or low antimicrobial activity against the four most common organisms: *Actinomyces*, *Viellonella*, *Eikenella*, and *Moraxella* species. In those few cases that are poorly controlled with this antibiotic protocol, the addition of metronidazole (Flagyl), 500 mg, three times daily for a 10-day course adds further control.

We have found that 88% of patients with intravenous bisphosphonate-induced osteonecrosis can be managed in a functional and pain-free state with this protocol and that only 5% are sufficiently nonresponsive or progress to a pathologic fracture that requires a partial jaw resection [25]. The remaining 7% of patients have succumbed to their cancer.

Oral bisphosphonate-induced osteonecrosis

Oral bisphosphonate-induced osteonecrosis differs from that caused by an intravenous bisphosphonate in several ways. It is statistically less likely (prevalence of approximately 0.015%) and it takes longer to develop because of slower accumulation in bone. This difference is offset by the estimated 14 million women taking oral bisphosphonates in the United States and another 8 million women in Europe and other countries. Its clinical expression is also less extensive (Fig. 9) and more responsive to surgery, and its risk of development can be assessed and stratified by a simple blood test [8,18]. The blood test is a morning fasting serum C-terminal telopeptide (CTX), which measures an octapeptide fragment released from type I bone collagen when an osteoclast resorbs bone [30]. It is an index of bone turnover, with lower values representing suppressed bone turnover and a reduced healing capability. We have stratified a risk level as follows values: values less than 100 pg/mL represent high risk, values between 100 pg/mL and 150 pg/mL represent moderate risk, and values more than 150 pg/mL represent minimal or no risk. It should be noted that normal values currently reported by laboratories performing the test were derived before bisphosphonates and are inaccurate, with too wide a range of normal.

Prevention of oral bisphosphonate-induced osteonecrosis before or during therapy

Prevention of oral bisphosphonate-induced osteonecrosis encompasses the same dental principles as those discussed in the section on intravenous bisphosphonate-induced osteonecrosis.

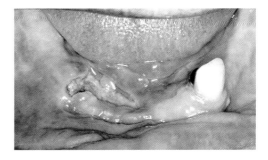

Fig. 9. Oral bisphosphonate-induced osteonecrosis is usually less extensive than intravenous bisphosphonate-induced osteonecrosis.

Dental practitioners must be sure to elicit the precise drug, its dose, its frequency and duration of therapy, and concomitant diseases and medications in their medical histories. This information is important because the limited absorption of bisphosphonates via the oral route extends the minimal risk period to the first 3 years of continuous use. Use of Fosamax also has a greater number of reported cases to date than Actonel for reasons that remain unclear at this time [8,18]. Concomitant diseases and medications are important because prednisone and methotrexate—both of which are commonly used to treat autoimmune diseases, such as rheumatoid arthritis and systemic lupus erythematosus—enhance the risk for BIONJ and increase its severity and reduce its rate of response to drug discontinuation. Use of ranitidine and other H_2 blocking drugs also may increase the risk for oral BIONJ because of increased absorption of the bisphosphonate.

It is hoped that as the medical community becomes more aware of BIONJ from oral bisphosphonates they will readily refer patients to qualified dentists for evaluation and the same preventive measures as were described for intravenous bisphosphonate-induced osteonecrosis. It is incumbent upon the dental profession to open greater lines of communication to the medical profession than currently exist and for dental professionals not to be intimated by a patient's bisphosphonate risk. An understanding of the CTX test and the treatment guidelines offered in this article should alleviate any reticence to treat these patients and actually encourage treatment that has been shown to prevent and resolve this form of BIONJ.

An individual patient who is referred by a physician or who presents for a dental evaluation and has taken an oral bisphosphonate for less than 3 years can be treated as any other patient. Although CTX testing may be useful as a reference, it is not necessary with this relatively short duration of bisphosphonate use. Within this 3-year window of relatively safe opportunity, however, the dental team should remove nonrestorable teeth and accomplish any indicated periodontal surgeries, preferably early in the treatment plan, followed by any other indicated noninvasive procedures that work toward the goal of optimum dental health and long-term stability.

For patients who report oral bisphosphonate use exceeding 3 years, palliation of pain and infection and obtaining a CTX test are recommended. Values more than 150 pg/mL indicate that invasive procedures can be accomplished with anticipation of healing; however, values less than 150 pg/mL indicate a potential healing compromise that may result in osteonecrosis. The dentist should consult with the prescribing physician to request a temporary discontinuation of the oral bisphosphonate, which is known as a "drug holiday." Most physicians accept a drug holiday because several recent studies have shown that even extended drug holidays from oral bisphosphonates of up to 5 years have not resulted in an increased incidence of osteoporosis-related fractures [31,32]. The dentist should not take it upon himself or herself to discontinue the oral bisphosphonate prescribed by another health care provider. Should the physician be reluctant to begin a drug holiday, substitute drugs with proven efficacy for preventing fractures caused by osteoporosis may be suggested, including raloxifene (Evista), recombinant human 1-34 parathyroid hormone (Forteo), and salmon calcitonin (Miacalcin), none of which is a bisphosphonate.

A drug holiday of 4 to 6 months is recommended before a repeat CTX test. We have observed that the CTX value rises approximately 20 pg/mL to 25 pg/mL but may be somewhat slower in patients who have received prednisone or methotrexate or have taken an oral bisphosphonate for 7 or more years.

Treatment of established oral bisphosphonate-induced osteonecrosis

The treatment goals for oral BIONJ are different from intravenous BIONJ because it is more curable. The first goal in treatment is initial intermediate-term palliation followed by either spontaneous resolution or resolution gained by débridement surgery. Patients also should be informed of the nature and natural course of their disease, however. They should be informed that osteoporosis is a serious disease, that osteoporosis-related fractures of the vertebrae and femur can be painful and disabling, and that their bisphosphonate therapy to date has been beneficial in preventing these fractures. They also should be informed that you will send a consultation report to the prescribing physician and that they should see their physician frequently to monitor their osteopenia/osteoporosis.

The initial therapy for oral bisphosphonate-induced osteonecrosis is prevention of pain with the use of 0.12% chlorhexidine 30-mL swish-and-spit

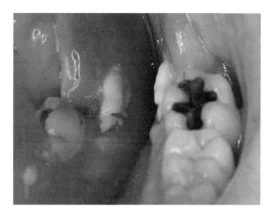

Fig. 10. Exposed bone in a patient who took Fosamax for 4.2 years and had a CTX value of 72 pg/mL.

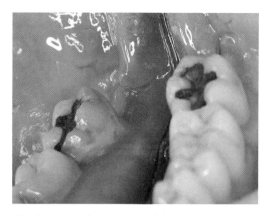

Fig. 11. Resolution of exposed bone without surgery after a drug holiday of 9 months as the CTX value rose to 212 pg/mL.

regimen three times daily, a CTX test, and a drug holiday requested if the patient is still taking the bisphosphonate. If pain or infection is present, the antibiotic regimens discussed in the section on management of intravenous bisphosphonate-induced osteonecrosis are indicated. The drug holiday should be followed for 6 months, at which time repeat CTX test results should be obtained. We have found that 40% of oral BIONJ cases resolve in this 6-month period without débridement in parallel to the CTX values rising to more than 150 pg/mL (Figs. 10 and 11). The remaining 60% of cases show clinical and radiographic signs of improvement, such as loosening or separation of the necrotic bone from adjacent healthy bone or a radiographic involucrum separating a sequestrum from adjacent bone as the CTX values increase (Figs. 12–14). At that time,

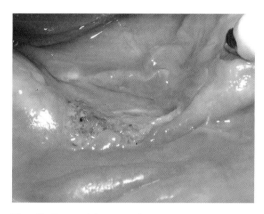

Fig. 12. Exposed bone (BIONJ) due to 6.0 years of Fosamax. CTX value was 55 pg/mL.

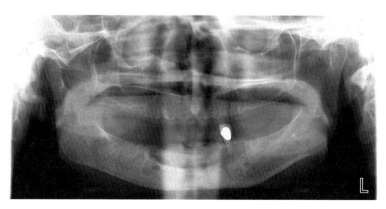

Fig. 13. Involucrum separates necrotic alveolar bone from viable bone during a drug holiday of 6 months and a CTX value that rose to 243 pg/mL.

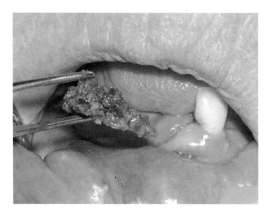

Fig. 14. Removal of sequestrum separated from viable bone eventuated into healed mucosa without further exposed bone.

local office-based sequestration/débridement with a primary closure can resolve the osteonecrosis. This result has been the case in all oral BIONJ cases except an advanced presentation of extensive osteonecrosis after 10.2 years of Fosamax therapy that required resection and titanium plate reconstruction (Figs. 15–18). To date we have resolved all 40 cases of osteonecrosis using this CTX-guided protocol. Follow-up on these patients has shown no recurrences provided that the CTX values are kept above the 150 pg/mL level by the prescribing physician using incremental drug schedules or alternative osteoporosis drugs.

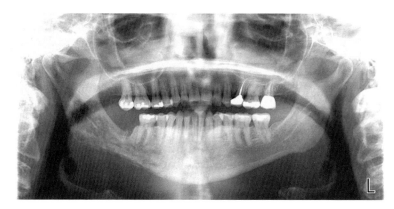

Fig. 15. Extensive bone necrosis caused by 10.2 years of steady Fosamax use.

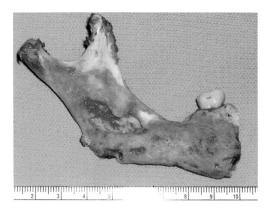

Fig. 16. Resection of hemimandible required because of extensive necrosis.

Summary

BIONJ is the correct term for this real drug complication that most dental practitioners face. All nitrogen-containing bisphosphonates pose a risk, which is related to the route of administration, the potency of the bisphosphonate, and the duration of use. Although intravenous BIONJ is mostly permanent, most cases can be prevented or managed if they develop, with only a few cases requiring resection for resolution. Oral BIONJ cases also can be prevented with knowledge of the risk level related to the duration of use and the CTX blood test results. Most cases can be resolved with a drug holiday either spontaneously or via straightforward débridement.

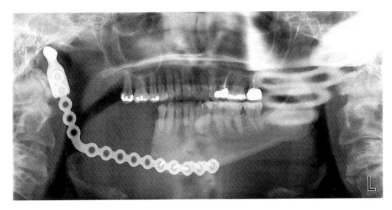

Fig. 17. Titanium plate reconstruction is able to replace bone resected because of BIONJ.

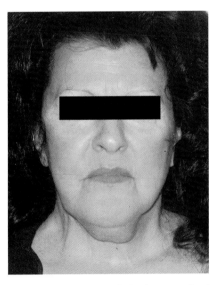

Fig. 18. Despite a hemimandibular jaw resection inclusive of the condyle, resolution of the BIONJ and maintenance of facial form can be achieved.

References

[1] Berenson JR, Rosen LS, Howell A, et al. Zoledronic acid reduces skeletal-related events in patients with osteolytic metastases: a double-blind, randomized, dose response study. Cancer 2001;91:1191–200.

[2] Major P. The use of zoledronic acid, a novel, highly potent bisphosphonate for the treatment of hypercalcemia of malignancy. Oncologist 2002;7:481–91.

[3] Cremers S, Sparidans R, Hartigh JD, et al. A pharmacokinetic and pharmacodynamic model for intravenous bisphosphonate (Pamidronate) in osteoporosis. Eur J Clin Pharmacol 2002;57:883–90.

[4] Jeffcoat MK. Safety of oral bisphosphonates: controlled studies on alveolar bone. Int J Oral Maxillofac Implants 2005;21:349–53.

[5] Santini D, Vespasianni GU, Vencenzi B, et al. The antineoplastic role of bisphosphonates from basic research to clinical evidence. Ann Oncol 2003;14: 1468–76.

[6] Odvina CV, Zerwelch JE, Sudhaker R, et al. Severely suppressed bone turnover: a potential complication of alendronate therapy. J Clin Endocrinol Metab 2005;90:1294–301.

[7] Adami S, Isaia G, Luisetto G, et al. Fracture incidence and characterization in patients on osteoporosis treatment: the ICARO study. J Bone Miner Res 2006;21:1565–70.

[8] Marx RE, Cillo JE, Ulloa JJ. Oral bisphosphonate induced osteonecrosis: risk factors, prediction of risk using serum CTX testing, prevention, and treatment, in press.

[9] Marx RE. Pamidronate (Aredia) and zoledronate (Zometa) induced avascular necrosis of the jaws: a growing epidemic. J Oral Maxillofac Surg 2003; 61:1115–7.

[10] Terasoff P, Csermak K. Avascular necrosis of the jaws: risk factors in metastatic cancer patients. J Oral Maxillofac Surg 2003;61:1238–9.

[11] Ruggerio SI, Mekrotia B, Engroff SI. Osteonecrosis of the jaws associated with the use of bisphosphonates: a review of 633 cases. J Oral Maxillofac Surg 2004;62:527–31.

[12] Migliorati CA. Bisphosphonates and oral cavity avascular bone necrosis. J Clin Oncol 2003;21: 4253–9.

[13] Migliorati CA, Casiglin J, Epstein J, et al. Managing the care of patients with bisphosphonate-associated osteonecrosis. J Am Dent Assoc 2005;136:1658–68.

[14] Markiewicz MR, Magarrne JE III, Campbell JH, et al. Bisphosphonate associated osteonecrosis of the jaws: a review of current knowledge. J Am Dent Assoc 2005;136:1669–74.

[15] Melo MD, Obeid G. Osteonecrosis of the jaws in patients with a history of receiving bisphosphonate therapy: strategies for prevention and early recognition. J Am Dent Assoc 2005;136:1675–81.

[16] Hoff A. Expert panel recommendation for prevention, diagnosis, and treatment of osteonecrosis of the jaws. Oncology Drug Advisory Committee Meeting. East Hanover, NJ, Novartis, March 4, 2005.

[17] Bamias A, Kastritis E, Bamia C, et al. Osteonecrosis of the jaw in cancer after treatment with bisphosphonates: incidence and risk factors. J Clin Oncol 2005; 23:8580–7.

[18] Marx RE, editor. Oral and intravenous bisphosphonate-induced osteonecrosis of the jaws: history, etiology, prevention, and treatment. Hanover Park (IL): Quintessence Publsihing; 2006.

[19] Widler L, Knut JA, Marcus A, et al. Highly potent germinal bisphosphonates: from pamidronate disoduim (Aredia) to zoledronic acid (Zometa). J Med Chem 2002;45:3721–38.

[20] Van Beek Er, Lowick CWGM, Papapoulous SE. Bisphosphonates suppress bone resorption by a direct effect on early osteoclast precursors without affecting the osteoclastogenic capacity of osteogenic cells: the role of protein geranylation in the action of nitrogen containing bisphosphonates on osteoclast precursors. Bone 2002;30:64–70.

[21] Glowacki J. Bisphosphonates and bone. Orthopedic Journal at Harvard Medical School 2005;7: 64–7.

[22] Russell RGA, Croucher PI, Rogers MJ. Bisphosphonates: pharmacology, mechanisms of action and clinical uses. Osteoporos Int 1999; 9(Suppl 2):S66–80.

[23] American Association Oral Maxillofacial Surgeons. Position paper on bisphosphonate-related osteonecrosis of the jaws. J Oral Maxillofac Surg 2007;65(3): 369–76.

[24] Marx RE, Sawatari Y, Fortin M, et al. Bisphosphonate induced exposed bone (osteonecrosis/osteopetrosis) of the jaws: risk factors, recognition, prevention, and treatment. J Oral Maxillofac Surg 2005;63:1567–75.

[25] Mellal A, Wiskott HW, Botsis J, et al. Stimulating effect of implant loading on surrounding bone: comparison in of three numerical models and validation by in vivo data. Clin Oral Implants Res 2004;15: 239–48.

[26] Cauley LK, Mohutic RM. Mediators of periodontal osseous destruction and remodeling: principles and complications for diagnosis and therapy. J Periodontol 2002;73:1377–91.

[27] Dixon RB, Trickler ND, Garetto LP. Bone turnover in elderly canine mandible and tibia. J Dent Res (JADR abstracts) 1997;76:2579.

[28] Lyns KP, Jensen JL. Dental lesions causing abnormalities on skeletal scientography. Clin Nucl Med 1979;4:509–12.

[29] Hellenstein JW, Marek CL. Bisphosphonate induced osteochemonecrosis of the jaws: an ounce of prevention may be worth a pound of care. Spec Care Dentist 2006;36:8–12.

[30] Rosen HN, Moses AC, Garber J, et al. Serum CTX: a new marker of bone resorption that shows treatment effect more often than other markers because of low coefficient of variability and large changes with bisphosphonate therapy. Calcif Tissue Int 2000;66:100–3.

[31] Black Dm, Schwartz AV, Enssrud KE, et al. Effects of continuing or stopping alendronate after 5 years of treatment: the fracture intervention trial long term extension (FLEX). A randomized trial. JAMA 2006;296:2927–38.

[32] Bone HQ, Hosking D, Devogelar J-P, et al. Ten years experience with alendronate for osteoporosis in postmenopausal women. N Engl J Med 2004; 350:1189–99.

ELSEVIER
SAUNDERS

Oral Maxillofacial Surg Clin N Am 19 (2007) 499–512

**ORAL AND
MAXILLOFACIAL
SURGERY CLINICS**
of North America

Bone Replacement Grafts for the Treatment of Periodontal Intrabony Defects

Philip J. Hanes, DDS, MS

*Department of Periodontics, Medical College of Georgia, School of Dentistry,
1459 Laney Walker Boulevard, Augusta, GA 30912–1220, USA*

An ultimate goal of periodontal therapy is the regeneration of periodontal supporting tissues that have been lost as a consequence of periodontitis. Wound healing studies have shown that removal of local bacterial etiology by surgical or nonsurgical therapies results in a resolution of inflammation and an improvement in the clinical signs of periodontitis, but it does not result in the regeneration of a periodontal connective tissue attachment [1,2]. Varying amounts of periodontal regeneration have been reported, however, when surgical therapy has included techniques of osseous grafting, guided tissue regeneration (GTR), or growth or amelogenin-type factors [3]. According to the American Academy of Periodontology 2005 position paper, "periodontal regeneration is defined histologically as regeneration of the tooth's supporting tissues, including alveolar bone, periodontal ligament, and cementum over a previously diseased root surface" [3]. The limitations inherent in current methods of periodontal examination make it impossible for clinicians to determine whether the healing responses they observe in their patients after various so-called "regenerative treatments" actually results in true histologic periodontal regeneration. After nonsurgical and surgical periodontal therapy, the improvements that occur in the clinical signs of periodontitis, such as reduced gingival inflammation and bleeding, reductions in periodontal probing depths, gains in probing attachment levels, and improvements in the architecture of intrabony defects as depicted on radiographs, are all

clinical findings that would be expected to occur with or without true periodontal regeneration [4].

To evaluate their attempts at periodontal regeneration, clinicians depend on clinical observations such as reduced probing depths, improvements in probing attachment levels, and bone fill. Bone fill is the clinical restoration of bone tissue in a treated periodontal defect [3]. Quantity of bone fill is usually determined by comparisons of pre- and posttreatment radiographs, bone-sounding with a periodontal probe, or surgical re-entry. As with other clinical means of evaluating periodontal healing responses, bone fill does not address the presence or absence of histologic evidence of true periodontal regeneration. The purpose of this article is to summarize the current information supporting the use of osseous grafting techniques to accomplish periodontal regeneration, focusing on the amount of bone fill that has been reported with various bone replacement grafting materials.

Attempts to regenerate bone by the placement of bone substitutes into periodontal intrabony defects have been reported since the late nineteenth century [5]. Although the rationale for such early attempts at periodontal regeneration was speculative at best, by the latter half of the twentieth century researchers showed that demineralized bone contained bone morphogenetic proteins that could induce bone formation [6,7] and that bone marrow cells in grafts of cancellous bone and marrow could induce new bone formation [8]. Many case series studies and controlled clinical trials conducted over the last half-century testing various types of bone replacement graft materials have shown positive clinical benefits associated with the treatment of periodontal

E-mail address: phanes@mail.mcg.edu

intrabony defects with these agents [9]. Currently, bone replacement grafts, including autografts, allografts, xenografts, and alloplasts, are the most widely used treatments for the regeneration of periodontal supporting tissues lost as a consequence of periodontitis.

Autogenous bone replacement grafts

Autogenous grafts of cortical or cancellous bone for the treatment of periodontal defects have been harvested from extra- and intraoral donor sites. In a series of case reports from the early 1970s, autogenous and allogenous grafts of cancellous bone and marrow from the posterior iliac crest were shown to have a marked ability to induce new bone formation in periodontal defects. They resulted in closure of seven of eight furcations, complete osseous fill of 11 of 21 one-wall defects and 33 of 33 two-wall defects, mean bone fill in intrabony defects exceeding 3 mm, and more than 2 mm of crestal bone apposition [10,11]. Although these studies demonstrated a marked potential for osseous regeneration in periodontal defects that are generally not considered to be amenable to periodontal regenerative therapy, including furcations, one-wall defects, and crestal bone loss, this type of osseous grafting is not routine in clinical periodontics because of the morbidity of the procedure for harvesting the donor bone and the incidence of root resorption reported with this technique [8,11,12]. A more common practice in contemporary periodontics involves the use of autogenous bone harvested from intraoral donor sites. In a case series, Hiatt and Schallhorn [13] used autogenous bone replacement grafts obtained from the maxillary tuberosity, extraction sockets, or edentulous ridges for the treatment of one-, two-, and three-wall defects. They reported a mean bone fill of 3.44 mm, which was more than 50% of the original defect depth [13]. Ellegaard and Löe [14] used autogenous bone replacement grafts of cancellous and cortical bone from edentulous intraoral sites for the treatment of two- and three-wall intrabony defects and reported complete osseous regeneration in 72% of three-wall and 45% of two-wall defects.

The best results with osseous grafting techniques occurred with the treatment of maxillary or mandibular anterior teeth, and the poorest results occurred in maxillary posterior teeth. In addition to the aforementioned case series studies, at least three controlled clinical trials have compared intraoral autogenous bone replacement grafts with a control treatment of open flap débridement for the treatment of intrabony periodontal defects (Table 1). Carraro and colleagues [15] compared the treatment of intrabony defects with intraoral autogenous cancellous bone replacement grafts to surgical débridement and reported 2.88 mm bone fill at grafted sites compared with 2.18 mm at control sites. Another form of intraoral autogenous bone replacement graft is the osseous coagulum–bone blend graft, which is an autogenous graft of bone shavings and blood clot that are collected during osseous recontouring procedures. Froum and colleagues [16,17] reported 70% fill of intrabony defects treated with osseous coagulum–bone blend compared with 22% fill at sites treated by débridement alone.

A more recent study by Renvert and colleagues [18] reported only 1.2 mm or approximately 25% bone fill of osseous defects after citric acid conditioning of root surfaces and placement of maxillary tuberosity bone replacement grafts. This amount of bone fill was similar to the amount

Table 1
Controlled clinical trials of autogenous bone replacement grafts for the treatment of intrabony defects

| Study | Graft material | Subject (n) | Defect (n) | Osseous regeneration | |
				Graft	Débridement
Carraro et al [15]	Oral auto	55	Oral auto = 56	95% ≥1mm[a]	82% ≥1mm[a]
			Control = 44		
Froum et al [17]	Oral auto- osseous coagulum	28	Oral auto = 37	70.6%[b]	21.8%[b]
			Control = 38		
Renvert et al [18]	Oral auto	19	Oral auto = 25	1.2 mm[c]	0.8 mm[c]
			Control = 28		

[a] Percentage of sites with ≥1 mm bone fill.
[b] Percentage resolution of original defect size.
[c] Mean amount of bone fill as measured from base of defect in relation to cementoenamel junction.

they observed at sites treated by surgical débridement and citric acid conditioning without the bone replacement graft. The less-than-optimal amount of bone regeneration reported in studies such as those by Renvert and colleagues after the use of autogenous bone grafts from the maxillary tuberosity may have been related to the deficiency of hematopoietic marrow in autografts harvested from the maxillary tuberosity [19].

Osseous allografts

In response to the desire for an osseous grafting material that could be obtained in sufficient quantities to treat multiple periodontal defects without increasing the need for a second surgical site for harvesting the donor bone, investigators began testing the clinical response to allografts of bone for the treatment of periodontal defects. Shrad and Tussing [20] described a controlled clinical study that compared the treatment of multiple intrabony defects in six patients with either frozen allografts of iliac bone and marrow or surgical débridement of the defects (Table 2). They reported a significantly greater 54.5% bone fill rate at grafted sites compared with 33.4% at control sites. Because of the infectious and immunologic risks associated with transplants and grafts of fresh or frozen allografts, investigators began testing osseous allografts that were processed in various ways to reduce immunogenicity and the risk of infectious disease transmission. Mellonig and colleagues [21] described a case series in which 97 intrabony defects in 48 patients were treated with freeze-dried allografts of crushed cortical bone (FDBA). At surgical re-entry 1 year after treatment, they observed more than 50% bone fill in 64% and complete osseous regeneration in 24% of treated defects. In a similar fashion, Sepe and colleagues [22] reported more than 50% bone fill in 60% of 189 grafted defects in 97 patients. According to Sepe and colleagues, the amount of osseous regeneration observed at surgical re-entry was greater in three-wall defects than in two- or one-wall defects.

In a controlled clinical trial, Altiere and colleagues [23] compared the treatment of ten paired intrabony defects with either freeze-dried bone allograft or surgical débridement (see Table 2). At surgical re-entry 1 year after treatment, Altiere and colleagues also reported more than 50% bone fill in approximately 60% of defects treated with the FDBA. The same amount of bone fill also was observed in the control sites

treated only by surgical débridement, however. Blumenthal and Steinberg [24] compared the treatment of intrabony defects with either autolysed antigen-extracted allogeneic bone or surgical débridement and reported 50% or more resolution of defects in 50% of sites treated with the allogeneic bone graft compared with none of the control sites. In a similar fashion, Borghetti and colleagues [25] compared the treatment of intrabony defects with either cryopreserved cancellous bone allografts or surgical débridement and reported 59% resolution of grafted defects compared with 27% resolution of control sites. In general, allografts of freeze-dried bone have been shown to result in 50% to 60% resolution of intrabony periodontal defects as evaluated by surgical re-entry [26,27]. Histologic studies have shown that FDBA particles are eventually resorbed by 30 months after treatment, but histologic evidence supporting the regeneration of a periodontal attachment apparatus, including regenerated bone and periodontal ligament after the use of FDBA, is lacking [28].

In response to the work of Urist and others describing a bone-inductive potential for demineralized allograft bone, investigators began to study the ability of demineralized freeze-dried bone allografts (DFDBA) to regenerate bone. In a histologic study in guinea pigs comparing the osteogenic potential of FDBA, DFDBA, and autogenous bone blend–osseous coagulum grafts, DFDBA had the greatest osteogenic potential, whereas FDBA had the least [29]. To test the osteogenic potential of DFDBA in humans, Quintero and colleagues [30] described a case series in which intrabony defects were treated with DFDBA and examined by surgical re-entry 6 months after treatment. The amount of osseous regeneration observed overall was approximately 65% of the original defect or 2.4 mm of vertical bone height, as measured from the base of the defect. In addition to this case series, several controlled clinical trials have compared the treatment of periodontal intrabony defects with DFDBA to surgical débridement (see Table 2). In an early clinical trial, Pearson and colleagues [31] compared DFDBA osseous grafting of 16 intrabony defects to surgical débridement of 6 defects in a total of seven patients. Mean bone fill of 1.38 mm was reported for defects treated with the DFDBA compared with 0.33 mm for the defects treated by surgical débridement. In a controlled clinical trial that involved 11 patients, Mellonig [32] compared the treatment of 32 intrabony defects with

Table 2
Controlled clinical trials of osseous allografts for the treatment of intrabony defects

Study	Graft material	Subject (n)	Defect (n)	Osseous regeneration	
				Graft	Débridement
Schrad & Tussing [20]	Frozen iliac marrow allograft	6	Iliac Marrow = 23	54.5%[a]	33.4%[a]
			Control = 32		
Altiere et al [23]	FDBA	9	FDBA = 10	60% ≥50%[b]	60% ≥50%[b]
			Control = 10		
Blumenthal & Steinberg [24]	AAA	10	AAA = 14	50% ≥50%[b]	0% ≥50%[b]
			Control = 15		
Borghetti et al [25]	CCBA	10	CCBA = 16	59%[a]	27%[a]
			Control = 13		
Mabry et al [47]	FDBA + TTC FDBA	16	61 total	72.7%[a] 48.4%[a]	46.1%[a]
Brown et al [36]	DFDBA	16	DFDBA = 8	42%[a]	32%[a]
			Control = 8		
Flemmig et al [34]	DFDBA	14	DFDBA = 14	46.1%[a]	19.2%[a]
			Control = 14		
Masters et al [37]	DFDBA + TTC DFDBA	15	DFDBA + TTC = 15 DFDBA = 15	77.3%[a] 77.9%[a]	63.8%[a]
			Control = 15		
Meadows et al [33]	DFDBA	10	DFDBA = 10	65%[a]	11.2%[a]
			Control = 10		
Mellonig [32]	DFDBA	11	DFDBA = 32	64.7%[a]	37.8%[a]
			Control = 15		
Pearson et al [31]	DFDBA	7	DFDBA = 16	1.38 mm[c]	0.33 mm[c]
			Control = 6		
Yukna et al [35]	DFDBA	31	DFDBA = 31	51.4%[a]	40.3%[a]
			Control = 31		

Abbreviations: AAA, autolysed antigen-extracted allogeneic bone; CCBA, cryopreserved cancellous bone allograft; DFDBA, demineralized freeze-dried bone allograft; FDBA, freeze-dried bone allograft; TTC, tetracycline.

[a] Percentage resolution of original defect size.
[b] Percentage of sites with ≥50% resolution of original defect.
[c] Mean amount of bone fill as measured from base of defect in relation to cementoenamel junction.

DFDBA to that of surgical débridement in an additional 15 defects. He reported an overall 65% osseous regeneration in the DFDBA-treated defects compared with 38% in the sham-operated control group. Seventy-eight percent of defects treated with DFDBA had more than 50% osseous regeneration compared with 40% of sites treated by surgical débridement.

Meadows and colleagues [33] described a clinical trial comparing the treatment of intrabony defects with DFDBA, polylactic acid granules, and surgical débridement. Ten intrabony defects were treated in each group in a total of ten patients. At surgical re-entry 6 months after the bone replacement graft therapy, bone fill of 65% was observed at sites treated with DFDBA compared with 11.2% at control sites. In a long-term study, Flemmig and colleagues [34] treated 14 intrabony defects each in 14 patients with either DFDBA or surgical débridement and reported 46.1% bone fill at the sites treated with DFDBA compared with 19.2% bone fill at control sites. This amount of osseous regeneration was maintained over the 3-year follow-up period of the study. In a multicenter clinical trial, Yukna and colleagues [35] compared the treatment of intrabony defects with DFDBA, anorganic bovine-derived hydroxyapatite (HA) matrix plus P-15, and surgical débridement. An overall mean bone fill of 54% was reported for the sites treated with DFDBA compared with 40.3% at control sites. Brown and colleagues [36] described a clinical trial that compared the treatment of intrabony defects with DFDBA, calcium phosphate cement, or surgical débridement and reported a mean bone fill of 42% at sites treated with DFDBA compared with 32% for sited treated by surgical débridement.

Not unlike freeze-dried bone allografts, studies of DFDBA generally have reported resolution of periodontal intrabony defects in the range of 50% to 60%, with a few studies reporting defect resolution as high as 78% [37]. Unlike freeze-dried bone allografts, however, histologic evidence in humans documents the regeneration of a periodontal attachment apparatus, including regenerated bone and periodontal ligament, after the treatment of periodontal intrabony defects with DFDBA. In a series of controlled, human histologic studies, Bowers and colleagues [38–40] reported greater resolution of intrabony defects treated with DFDBA compared with surgical débridement. Regeneration of a periodontal attachment apparatus, including new bone and periodontal ligament, also occurred at sites treated with DFDBA, whereas a long junctional epithelium formed adjacent to exposed root surfaces at sites treated by surgical débridement [38,39].

The biologic rationale for the treatment of periodontal intrabony defects with DFDBA is based on the assumption that the demineralization of the allograft bone exposes bone morphogenetic proteins, which have been shown to be capable of inducing or enhancing bone regeneration [6,7,41]. In terms of the overall resolution of the intrabony defect, however, clinical studies to date have not shown a superiority of DFDBA over FDBA. Most studies have reported an overall 50% to 60% defect resolution with DFDBA and FDBA. Rummelhart and colleagues [42] did a direct clinical comparison of DFDBA and FDBA in the treatment of paired intrabony defects and observed no differences between the two graft materials in terms of defect resolution at the 6-month surgical re-entry. Studies suggest that the reason for the failure of DFDBA to show a greater osseous regeneration potential is the insufficient amount of bone morphogenetic protein present in most commercially available preparations of DFDBA [43]. Such studies have shown that the amount of bone morphogenetic protein present in the DFDBA material varies widely among different commercial bone banks [44] and depends greatly on the age of the donor, with lower osteogenic activity noted in samples from older donors [45]. Despite these reported inconsistencies in the biologic activity of DFDBA obtained from different tissue banks, DFDBA is still considered to be an appropriate treatment modality for attempts to regenerate periodontal tissues lost as a consequence of periodontitis [46].

In an attempt to enhance the osteogenic potential of the graft material, some investigators have incorporated tetracycline into the reconstituted allograft bone at the time of graft placement. Mabry and colleagues [47] incorporated tetracycline powder into freeze-dried bone allografts at a ratio of 4:1 FDBA to tetracycline for the treatment of intrabony defects in adolescents with localized aggressive periodontitis. Greater defect resolution was reported with the addition of the tetracycline amounting to 72.7% bone fill compared with 48.4% at sites treated with FDBA alone and 46.1% with surgical débridement.

In contrast to the aforementioned study, Masters and colleagues [37] compared DFDBA alone with DFDBA plus tetracycline for the treatment of intrabony defects in chronic periodontitis and found no difference in defect resolution with the two treatment methods. Intrabony defects were treated with DFDBA, DFDBA plus 50 mg/mL tetracycline, or surgical débridement. A mean bone fill of 77.9% was reported for sites treated with DFDBA alone, 77.3% for sites treated with DFDBA plus tetracycline, and 63.8% for sites treated by surgical débridement. The reason for the disparate results in these two studies is unclear but may be related to the different periodontal diagnoses that were treated in the two studies—localized aggressive periodontitis versus chronic periodontitis—or to the different ages of the two study populations. Currently no compelling evidence supports the incorporation of antibiotics into bone replacement grafts such as DFDBA to enhance the osseous regeneration obtained with the procedure. In a recent meta-analysis, however, systemic antibiotics administered in conjunction with surgical and nonsurgical periodontal therapy have been shown to provide a significant—albeit small—additional clinical benefit to mechanical therapy alone in terms of an additional 0.45 mm of probing attachment gain [48]

It may be possible to enhance the amount of bone fill obtained with bone replacement grafts such as DFDBA by combining regenerative therapies. A recent meta-analysis of four clinical trials showed a modest but insignificant trend for greater bone fill with combined therapy of bone replacement grafts plus GTR compared with treatment with bone replacement grafts alone [9]. Gurinsky and colleagues [49] also compared the treatment of defects with either DFDBA plus enamel matrix derivative (EMD) or EMD alone and reported 74.9% bone fill at sites treated with DFDBA plus EMD compared with 55.3% at sites treated by EMD alone. The amount of bone fill reported with the DFDBA plus EMD treatment in this study is considerably greater than the 60% bone fill that most studies have reported with the use of DFDBA alone.

Various materials have been added to allograft materials to serve as carriers to make handling of the graft material easier. Matzenbacher and colleagues [50] tested the osteogenic potential of DFDBA mixed with a glycerol carrier in rat calvarial defects. They reported no differences in bone formation between defects treated with or without the glycerol carrier but indicated that the handling characteristics of the DFDBA were greatly enhanced by the glycerol preparation. Bender and colleagues [51] described a clinical trial testing DFDBA alone, DFDBA paste with 2% sodium hyaluronate, and DFDBA putty with 4% sodium hyaluronate and reported no difference in defect resolution between the groups at the 6-month surgical re-entry.

Alloplastic bone substitutes

Alloplastic bone substitutes are either synthetic graft materials or inert foreign bodies that are implanted into osseous defects. Alloplastic bone substitutes that are used to treat periodontal defects include nonporous HA, porous HA (PHA), porous HA cement (PHAc), beta tricalcium phosphate, polymethylmethacrylate (PMMA), and PMMA and hydroxyethylmethacrylate (HEMA) polymers, and bioactive glass.

Nonporous hydroxyapatite

Rabalais and colleagues [52] described a 6-month controlled clinical trial that compared the treatment of intrabony defects in 18 patients with either HA or surgical débridement (Table 3). Mean fill of 51.8% was reported for sites treated with the HA compared with 31.4% for control sites. In a total of 12 patients, Meffert and colleagues [53] compared the treatment of 16 defects with HA to that of 12 defects with surgical débridement and reported a mean bone fill of 66.9% at sites treated with HA compared with 9.9% at control sites. In a study of durapatite ceramic HA, Yukna and colleagues [54] reported mean bone fill of 43.7% at sites treated with HA compared with 29.9% at control sites.

Porous hydroxyapatite and porous hydroxyapatite cement

PHA is an analog of coral. The natural coral skeleton is a porous, resorbable material with a crystalline structure that is 98% calcium carbonate (CalCarb) [55]. PHA is an analog of the natural coral skeleton in which the CalCarb has undergone conversion to HA [56], which is a nonresorbable, biocompatible material with a structure of interconnected pores. Yukna [57] evaluated the osteogenic potential of alloplastic implants of resorbable, coralline CalCarb in periodontal defects in 20 patients (see Table 3). Forty defects were treated with the CalCarb graft material and an additional 39 defects were treated by surgical débridement. Mean bone fill of 67.7% was reported for sites treated with the CalCarb compared with 25.9% for control sites. Mora and Ouhayoun [55] compared coralline CalCarb, PHA, and surgical débridement for the treatment of ten intrabony defects each in ten patients. Mean bone fill of 57.4% was reported for sites treated with CalCarb compared with 58.1% for sites treated with PHA and 22.2% for control sites. Kim and colleagues [58] compared the treatment of intrabony defects with CalCarb, GTR plus CalCarb, GTR alone, and surgical débridement. Mean bone fill of 4 mm was reported for sites treated with the CalCarb graft compared with 0.5 mm for the surgical débridement sites. GTR barrier membranes did not enhance the amount of osseous regeneration in this study.

Kenney and colleagues [59] described a 6-month clinical trial comparing the treatment of 15 defects each with either PHA or surgical débridement. Mean bone fill of 3.53 mm was reported for sites treated with the PHA compared with 0.73 for control sites. Krejci and colleagues [60] compared the treatment of intrabony defects with HA, PHA, and surgical débridement. Mean bone fill of 38.2% was reported for sites treated with HA, compared with 23.8% for PHA sites and 9.0% for control sites. Brown and colleagues [36] compared the treatment of intrabony defects with PHAc, DFDBA, or surgical débridement. Mean bone fill of 29% was reported for sited treated with PHAc, compared with 42% for sites treated with DFDBA and 32% for control sites.

It may be possible to enhance the amount of bone fill that results from the treatment of intrabony defects with alloplastic bone substitutes by combining regenerative therapies. In a total of 18 patients, Kilic and colleagues [61] compared

Table 3
Controlled clinical trials of calcium carbonate, porous and nonporous hydroxyapatite alloplastic bone substitutes for the treatment of intrabony defects

| Study | Graft material | Subject (*n*) | Defect (*n*) | Osseous regeneration | |
				Graft	Débridement
Yukna [57]	CalCarb	20	CalCarb= 40 Control = 39	67.7%[a]	25.9%[a]
Kim et al [58]	CalCarb	31	CalCarb = 13 Control = 18	4.0 mm[b]	0.5 mm[b]
Mora & Ouhayoun [55]	Natural coral PHA	10	Natural coral = 10 PHA = 10 Control = 10	57.4%[a] 58.1%[a]	22.2%[a]
Kilic et al [61]	PHA	18	PHA = 10 Control = 10	23%[a]	15%[a]
Krejci et al [60]	Nonporous HA PHA	12	Nonporous HA = 12 PHA = 12 Control = 12	38.2%[a] 23.8%[a]	9%[a]
Brown et al [36]	PHA cement	16	HA cement = 16 Control = 8	29%[a]	32%[a]
Kenney et al [59]	PHA	25	PHA = 15 Control = 15	3.53 mm[b]	0.73 mm[b]
Meffert et al [53]	PHA	12	PHA = 16 Control = 12	66.9%[a]	9.9%[a]
Rabalais et al [52]	Nonporous HA	8	Nonporous HA = 88 Control = 60	51.8%[a]	31.4%[a]
Yukna et al [54]	Nonporous HA	13	Nonporous HA = 56 Control = 42	43.7%[a]	29.9%[a]

[a] Percentage resolution of original defect size.
[b] Mean amount of bone fill as measured from base of defect in relation to cementoenamel junction.

the treatment of ten defects each with (1) GTR using a nonresorbable expanded polytetrafluoroethylene (e-PTFE) barrier membrane, (2) GTR plus PHA–collagen graft, (3) PHA–collagen graft only, and (4) surgical débridement. Mean bone fill of 23% was reported for sited treated with PHA–collagen graft alone compared with 15% for sites treated by surgical débridement. The addition of the GTR barrier membrane increased the amount of bone fill with the PHA–collagen graft to 43%. In a more recent study, Okuda and colleagues [62] compared the treatment of osseous defects with either PHA alone or a combination of PHA plus platelet-rich plasma. The combination of PHA plus platelet-rich plasma resulted in 70.3% resolution of the original amount of clinical probing attachment loss compared with 45.5% at sites treated by PHA alone.

Polymethylmethacrylate and hydroxyethylmethacrylate polymers

PMMA/HEMA polymers for use as alloplastic bone substitutes are nonresorbable, microporous polymeric beads that are coated with calcium hydroxide (HTR polymer) [63]. Yukna [63] compared the treatment of intrabony defects with HTR polymer grafts to surgical débridement and reported mean bone fill of 60.8% at sites treated with the HTR polymer compared with 32.2% at control sites. Shahmiri and colleagues [64] described the treatment of intrabony defects in 15 patients with either HTR polymer grafts or surgical débridement (Table 4). Probing attachment loss improved by 38% at sites treated with the HTR polymer compared with 33% at control sites.

Bioactive glass

Bioactive glass is made from calcium salts, phosphate, sodium salts, and silicon. The addition of silicon allows for the formation of a silica gel layer over the bioactive glass particles, which promotes the formation of a hydroxycarbonate-apatite layer. This hydroxycarbonate-apatite layer facilitates the proliferation of osteoblasts and promotes bone formation [65]. Froum and colleagues [66] compared the treatment of intrabony defects with bioactive glass to surgical débridement and

Table 4
Controlled clinical trials of bioactive glass, polymethylmethacrylate/hydroxyethylmethacrylate polymeric alloplastic bone substitutes, and xenografts for the treatment of intrabony defects

Study	Graft material	Subject (n)	Defect (n)	Osseous regeneration Graft	Graft
Froum et al [66]	Bioactive glass	16	BG = 32 Control = 27	62.0%[a]	33.6%[a]
Ong et al [68]	Bioactive glass	14	BG = 14 Control = 14	23.1% >50%[b]	35.7% >50%[b]
Park et al [67]	Bioactive glass	38	BG = 21 Control = 17	2.8 mm[c]	1.3 mm[c]
Shahmiri et al [64]	PMMA/HEMA	15	PMMA/HEMA = 15 Control = 15	38%[d]	33%[d]
Yukna [63]	PMMA/HEMA	21	PMMA/HEMA = 71 Control = 68	60.8%[a]	32.2%[a]
Yukna et al [35]	Bovine xenograft + P-15	31	ABX/P-15 = 3 Control = 31	72.3%[a]	40.3%[a]

[a] Percentage resolution of original defect size.
[b] Percentage of sites with ≥50% resolution of original defect.
[c] Mean amount of bone fill as measured from base of defect in relation to cementoenamel junction.
[d] Percentage reduction of original amount of probing attachment loss.

reported mean bone fill of 62% at sites treated with the bioactive glass compared with 33.6% at control sites (see Table 4). Park and colleagues [67] compared the treatment of 21 intrabony defects with bioactive glass to that of 17 defects treated by surgical débridement. Bone sounding measurements 6 months after treatment showed a mean bone fill of 2.8 mm at sites treated with the bioactive glass compared with 1.3 mm at control sites. Ong and colleagues [68] also compared the treatment of intrabony defects with bioactive glass to surgical débridement. In contrast to the findings of Froum and colleagues and Park and colleagues, however, Ong and colleagues reported greater bone fill in control defects than in defects treated with the bioactive glass. Only 23.1% of sites treated with the bioactive glass had more than 50% defect fill compared with 35.7% of sites treated by surgical débridement.

Generally, the clinical results obtained after the treatment of intrabony defects with alloplastic bone substitutes is similar to that observed after treatment with DFDBA in terms of bone fill, pocket depth reductions, and probing attachment gains [26,69]. Unlike DFDBA, however, alloplastic bone substitutes have not been shown to result in histologic regeneration of the periodontal attachment apparatus. Most often, histologic studies have shown implants of alloplastic bone substitutes to be encapsulated by connective tissue with little or no bone formation associated with them [70–72].

Xenografts

Currently available xenografts for the treatment of periodontal defects include bovine-derived osseous grafting materials such as anorganic bovine bone (ABB) (Bio-Oss). Xenografts such as Bio-Oss are also referred to as anorganic bone because tissue processing methods generally remove all cells and proteinaceous material and leave behind a resorbable, mineralized bone scaffolding. Richardson and colleagues [73] compared the treatment of intrabony defects in 17 patients with either ABB or DFDBA. Fourteen defects were treated with DFDBA and 16 with ABB. Six months after treatment, mean bone fill at surgical re-entry was 58.1% in the sites treated with ABB compared with 67.7% at sites treated with DFDBA. ABB has been studied recently as a component of combined techniques to achieve periodontal and osseous regeneration. Paolantonio [74] described the treatment of 34 patients with either ABB plus a collagen membrane or GTR with the collagen membrane alone. Mean vertical bone gain in intrabony defects was 5.23 mm at sites treated with the combined technique compared with 3.82 at the sites treated with the GTR barrier alone [74].

Cortellini and Tonetti [75] compared the treatment of intrabony defects in 40 patients with four different regenerative techniques: (1) GTR with a nonresorbable barrier, (2) GTR with a resorbable barrier, (3) combined technique of ABB plus a resorbable barrier, and (4) EMD. They reported an equivalent resolution of the intrabony defect with all four techniques ranging from 88.2% to 92.1%. Resolution of the defects in this study, however, was determined on the basis of changes in clinical probing attachment levels. In another study of ABB combined with EMD, Velasquez-Plata and colleagues [76] reported 0.9 mm more bone fill with ABB plus EMD compared with EMD alone. This same group of investigators also compared the treatment of intrabony defects with either ABB plus EMD or ABB alone and reported an equivalent amount of bone fill with both techniques ranging from 63% to 67% [77]. These studies suggested that ABB plays a greater role in the hard tissue resolution of an intrabony defect than does EMD.

Yukna and colleagues [78] also tested a combination regenerative technique of ABB plus P-15 cell binding peptide comparing it to ABB alone. Mean defect fill of 72.9 % was reported for the sites treated with the combination therapy compared with 50.7% for sites treated with the xenograft alone. In a controlled clinical trial, Yukna and colleagues [35] compared the treatment of intrabony defects in 31 patients with (1) a combination of ABB plus cell-binding peptide P-15 (ABB + P-15), (2) DFDBA, or (3) surgical débridement (see Table 4). At surgical re-entry 6 months after treatment, mean bone fill of 72.3% was reported for sites treated with the ABB plus P-15, compared with 51.4% for sites treated with DFDBA and 40.3% for control sites. The evidence to support the use of xenografts for the treatment of periodontal defects is limited. Taken collectively, however, studies suggest that xenografts of ABB result in bone fill more than 50% and that the amount of bone fill obtained with this xenograft can be enhanced by adding P-15 cell-binding peptide to the ABB. These materials are more widely used for osseous grafting procedures for sinus lift procedures and ridge augmentation [79,80].

Factors that influence treatment success

In general, periodontal intrabony defects associated with furcations do not respond as favorably to regenerative therapy as do non–furcation-associated defects [13,17,27,47,66] Yukna and colleagues [81] compared the treatment of mandibular class II furcations with either an alloplastic bone substitute (bioactive glass) or GTR with a nonresorbable barrier. Mean horizontal furcation fill of only 31% to 32% was reported for both treatment groups, which is approximately one half the amount of bone fill reported by most studies of regenerative therapy in non–furcation-associated intrabony defects. Calongne and colleagues [82] compared the treatment of class II furcations with (1) PMMA/HEMA plus calcium hydroxide (HTR), (2) GTR with a nonresorbable barrier, or (3) HTR plus GTR. Mean horizontal furcation defect fill in the range of 19.4% to 37.5% was reported for the three treatments, each being considerably less favorable than the amount of bone fill that has been reported in previous studies of regenerative therapy at non-furcation sites. In contrast to these studies, Lamb and colleagues [83] described the treatment of class II furcations with combination therapy of DFDBA plus a nonresorbable GTR membrane and obtained more than 50% bone fill in 100% of 17 defects that had an intrabony component to the furcation defect.

Clinical and animal studies have demonstrated that the amount of periodontal regeneration obtained with any surgical technique is influenced by certain local and behavioral factors. For example, the morphology of the intrabony defect is particularly significant as studies have shown that attempts to obtain periodontal regeneration are more successful in deep-narrow defects than in shallow-wide defects [8,17,32]. Defects with two and three bony walls respond more favorably to treatment than do one-wall defects [17,22]. Attempts to obtain periodontal regeneration also are less successful in patients with poor oral hygiene [40,84], in smokers [84], and in patients who do not comply with periodontal maintenance therapy [85].

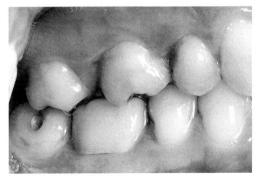

Fig. 1. Pretreatment view of maxillary right posterior sextant. Deep periodontal pockets and bleeding on probing were present interproximally between the first and second molars and the first molar and second premolar.

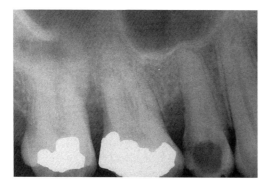

Fig. 2. Pretreatment radiograph of maxillary right posterior sextant. Intrabony defects were present interproximally between the first and second molars and the first molar and second premolar corresponding to the deep periodontal pockets in these sites. The second premolar also had a periapical radiolucency and clinically nonvital dental pulp.

Surgical technique

The surgical technique for the treatment of periodontal intrabony defects with bone replacement grafts is essentially the same regardless of the type of graft material being used. Incisions are designed to allow for primary closure of flaps to protect the graft site from infection and the graft material from displacement. Intrasulcular incisions are the common choice, with emphasis on preserving interdental tissue. Flaps are reflected

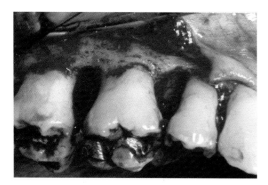

Fig. 3. After initial therapy that included oral hygiene instructions, scaling, and root planing and endodontic treatment of the maxillary second premolar, surgical therapy was performed. Full-thickness flaps were elevated facially and palatal, osseous defects were debrided of soft tissue, and root surfaces were thoroughly scaled and root planed. A two-wall intrabony defect was present between the first and second molars and a combination 1-, 2-, and 3-wall defect was present between the first molar and second premolar.

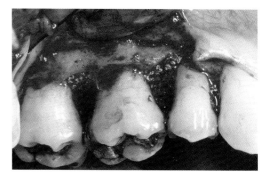

Fig. 4. Autogenous bone was harvested from a recent extraction site and packed into the apical portions of the intrabony defects. PHA was used to complete the filling of the defects to the level of the remaining crestal alveolar bone.

full thickness to expose the underlying osseous defects and allow access for thorough débridement of the defects and meticulous root planing (Figs. 1–3). Once the defect has been debrided of soft tissue and the tooth root surfaces thoroughly planed to remove all deposits of dental plaque and calculus, the bone replacement graft material is packed into the defect to fill the defect to the level of the remaining alveolar bone (Fig. 4). Flaps are closed and sutured for primary closure and complete coverage of the bone replacement graft. Sutures should be removed in 7 to 10 days. Postsurgical care should include twice-daily rinsing with 0.12% chlorhexidine gluconate for 2 weeks and gentle toothbrushing starting 1 week after the surgery. Systemic antibiotics may be prescribed for 7 to 10 days after the surgical procedure. Patients should be seen at intervals of 1 week, 2 weeks, and 4 weeks after surgery for

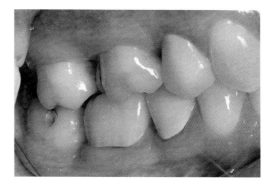

Fig. 5. One-year posttreatment view of the maxillary right posterior sextant. Periodontal probing depths have been reduced to 4 mm or less, and bleeding on probing has been resolved.

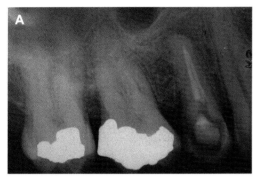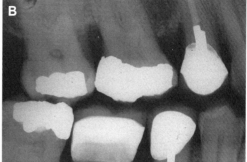

Fig. 6. One-year posttreatment radiographs show fill of intrabony defects (*A*) and a resolution of the angular bony defect between the first molar and second premolar (*B*).

supragingival plaque removal and then should be placed on a periodontal maintenance schedule at 3-month intervals. Figs. 5 and 6 show the clinical results of bone replacement graft therapy after 1 year of periodontal maintenance.

Summary

Bone replacement grafts, including autogenous grafts from intraoral donor sites, allografts, xenografts, and alloplastic bone substitutes, are the most widely used treatment modalities for the regeneration of periodontal osseous defects. Studies suggest a favorable clinical outcome with the use of these materials in terms of improvements in periodontal probing depths, probing attachment gains, and bone fill. Sites that are treated with bone replacement grafts have been shown to respond at least as well as surgical débridement of the defect alone and usually better—particularly in terms of bone fill. Meta-analysis from a recent evidence-based review indicated that bone replacement grafts increase bone level, reduce crestal bone loss, increase clinical attachment level, and reduce probing pocket depths when compared with open flap débridement procedures [9].

References

[1] Caton J, Zander HA. Osseous repair of an infrabony pocket without new attachment of connective tissue. J Clin Periodontol 1976;3:54–8.

[2] Caton J, Nyman S, Zander H. Histometric evaluation of periodontal surgery. II. Connective tissue attachment levels after four regenerative procedures. J Clin Periodontol 1980;7:224–31.

[3] American Academy of Periodontology. Periodontal regeneration [position paper]. J Periodontol 2005;76: 1601–22.

[4] Polson AM, Heijl LC. Osseous repair in infrabony periodontal defects. J Clin Periodontol 1978;5: 13–23.

[5] Senn N. On the healing of aseptic bone cavities by implantation of antiseptic decalcified bone. Am J Med Sci 1889;98:219.

[6] Urist MR, Dowell TA. The inductive substratum for osteogenesis in pellets of particulate bone matrix. Clin Orthop 1968;61:61–78.

[7] Urist MR, Strates BS. Bone morphogenetic protein. J Dent Res 1971;50:1392–406.

[8] Dragoo MR, Sullivan HC. A clinical and histological evaluation of autogenous iliac bone grafts in humans. I. Wound healing 2 to 8 months. J Periodontol 1973;44:599–613.

[9] Reynolds MA, Aichelmann-Reidy ME, Branch-Mays GL, et al. The efficacy of bone replacement grafts in the treatment of periodontal osseous defects: a systematic review. Ann Periodontol 2003;8: 227–65.

[10] Schallhorn RG, Hiatt WH, Boyce W. Iliac transplants in periodontal therapy. J Periodontol 1970; 41:566–80.

[11] Schallhorn RG, Hiatt WH. Human allografts of iliac cancellous bone and marrow in periodontal osseous defects. II. Clinical observations. J Periodontol 1972; 43:67–81.

[12] Burnette EW Jr. Fate of an iliac crest graft. J Periodontol 1972;43:88–90.

[13] Hiatt WH, Schallhorn RG. Intraoral transplants of cancellous bone and marrow in periodontal lesions. J Periodontol 1973;44:192–208.

[14] Ellegaard B, Löe H. New attachment of periodontal tissues after treatment of intrabony lesions. J Periodontol 1971;42:648–52.

[15] Carraro JJ, Sznajder N, Alonso CA. Intraoral cancellous bone autografts in the treatment of infrabony pockets. J Clin Periodontol 1976;3: 104–9.

[16] Froum SJ, Thaler R, Scopp IW, et al. Osseous auto-grafts. II. Histological responses to osseous coagulum bone blend grafts. J Periodontol 1975;46: 656–61.

[17] Froum SJ, Ortiz M, Witkin RT, et al. Osseous auto-grafts. III. Comparison of osseous coagulum-bone blend implants with open curettage. J Periodontol 1976;47:287–94.

[18] Renvert S, Garrett S, Schallhorn RG, et al. Healing after treatment of periodontal intraosseous defects. III. Effect of osseous grafting and citric acid conditioning. J Clin Periodontol 1985;12:441–55.

[19] Kucaba WJ, Simpson DM. Incidence and distribution of hematopoietic marrow in human maxillary tuberosity [abstract 265]. J Dent Res 1978;57:141.

[20] Schrad SC, Tussing GJ. Human allografts of iliac bone and marrow in periodontal osseous defects. J Periodontol 1986;57:205–10.

[21] Mellonig JT, Bowers GM, Bright RW, et al. Clinical evaluation of freeze-dried bone allografts in peri-odontal osseous defects. J Periodontol 1976;47: 125–31.

[22] Sepe WW, Bowers GM, Lawrence JJ, et al. Clinical evaluation of freeze-dried bone allografts in peri-odontal osseous defects: part II. J Periodontol 1978;49:9–14.

[23] Altiere ET, Reeve CM, Sheridan PJ. Lyophillized bone allografts in periodontal intraosseous defects. J Periodontol 1979;50:510–9.

[24] Blumenthal N, Steinberg J. The use of collagen membrane barriers in conjunction with combined demineralized bone-collagen implants in human infrabony defects. J Periodontol 1990;61:319–27.

[25] Borghetti A, Novakovitch G, Louise F, et al. Cryopreserved cancellous bone allograft in periodontal intraosseous defects. J Periodontol 1993;64: 128–32.

[26] Evans GH, Yukna RA, Sepe WW, et al. Effect of various graft materials with tetracycline in localized juvenile periodontitis. J Periodontol 1989;60:491–7.

[27] Barnett JD, Mellonig JT, Gray JL, et al. Comparison of freeze-dried bone allograft and porous hydroxyapatite in human periodontal defects. J Periodontol 1989;60:231–7.

[28] Froum SJ. Human histologic evaluation of HTR polymer and freeze-dried bone allograft: a case report. J Clin Periodontol 1996;23:615–20.

[29] Mellonig JT, Bowers GM, Bailey RC. Comparison of bone graft materials. Part I. New bone formation with autografts and allografts determined by strontium-85. J Periodontol 1981;52:291–6.

[30] Quintero G, Mellonig JT, Gambill VM, et al. A six-month clinical evaluation of decalcified freeze-dried bone allografts in periodontal osseous defects. J Periodontol 1982;53:726–30.

[31] Pearson GE, Rosen S, Deporter DA. Preliminary observations on the usefulness of a decalcified, freeze-dried cancellous bone allograft material in periodontal surgery. J Periodontol 1981;52:55–9.

[32] Mellonig JT. Decalcified freeze-dried bone allograft as an implant material in human periodontal defects. Int J Periodontics Restorative Dent 1984;6: 40–55.

[33] Meadows CL, Gher ME, Quintero G, et al. A comparison of polylactic acid granules and decalcified freeze-dried bone allograft in human periodontal osseous defects. J Periodontol 1993;64:103–9.

[34] Flemmig TF, Ehmke B, Bolz K, et al. Long-term maintenance of alveolar bone gain after implantation of autolyzed, antigen-extracted, allogenic bone in periodontal intraosseous defects. J Periodontol 1998;69:47–53.

[35] Yukna RA, Callan DP, Krauser JT, et al. Multicenter clinical evaluation of combination anorganic bovine-derived hydroxyapatite matrix (ABM)/cell binding peptide (P-15) as a bone replacement graft material in human periodontal osseous defects: 6-month results. J Periodontol 1998;69:655–63.

[36] Brown GD, Mealey BL, Nummikoski PV, et al. Hydroxyapatite cement implant for regeneration of periodontal osseous defects in humans. J Periodontol 1998;69:146–57.

[37] Masters LB, Mellonig JT, Brunsvold MA, et al. A clinical evaluation of demineralized freeze-dried bone allograft in combination with tetracycline in the treatment of periodontal osseous defects. J Periodontol 1996;67:770–81.

[38] Bowers GM, Chadroff B, Carnevale R, et al. Histologic evaluation of new attachment apparatus formation in humans. Part I. J Periodontol 1989;60: 664–74.

[39] Bowers GM, Chadroff B, Carnevale R, et al. Histologic evaluation of new attachment apparatus formation in humans. Part II. J Periodontol 1989;60: 675–82.

[40] Bowers GM, Chadroff B, Carnevale R, et al. Histologic evaluation of new attachment apparatus formation in humans. Part III. J Periodontol 1989;60: 683–93.

[41] Schwartz Z, Somers A, Mellonig JT, et al. Addition of human recombinant bone morphogenetic protein-2 to inactive commercial human demineralized freeze-dried bone allograft makes an effective composite bone inductive implant material. J Periodontol 1998;69:1337–45.

[42] Rummelhart JM, Mellonig JT, Gray JL, et al. A comparison of freeze-dried bone allograft and demineralized freeze-dried bone allograft in human periodontal osseous defects. J Periodontol 1989;60: 655–63.

[43] Shigeyama Y, D'Errico JA, Stone R, et al. Commercially-prepared allograft material has biological activity in vitro. J Periodontol 1995;66: 478–87.

[44] Becker W, Urist MR, Tucker LM, et al. Human demineralized freeze-dried bone: inadequate induced bone formation in athymic mice. A preliminary report. J Periodontol 1995;66:822–8.

[45] Schwartz Z, Somers A, Mellonig JT, et al. Ability of commercial demineralized freeze-dried bone allograft to induce new bone formation is dependent on donor age but not gender. J Periodontol 1998;69: 470–8.

[46] American Academy of Periodontology. Tissue banking of bone allografts used in periodontal regeneration [position paper]. J Periodontol 2001;72: 834–8.

[47] Mabry TW, Yukna RA, Sepe WW. Freeze-dried bone allografts combined with tetracycline in the treatment of juvenile periodontitis. J Periodontol 1985;56:74–81.

[48] Haffajee AD, Socransky SS, Gunsolley JC. Systemic anti-infective periodontal therapy: a systematic review. Ann Periodontol 2003;8:115–81.

[49] Gurinsky BS, Mills MP, Mellonig JT. Clinical evaluation of demineralized freeze-dried bone allograft and enamel matrix derivative versus enamel matrix derivative alone for the treatment of periodontal osseous defects in humans. J Periodontol 2004;75: 1309–18.

[50] Matzenbacher SA, Mailhot JM, McPherson JC, et al. In vivo effectiveness of a glycerol-compounded demineralized freeze-dried bone xenograft in the rat calvarium. J Periodontol 2003;74:1641–6.

[51] Bender SA, Rogalski JB, Mills MP, et al. Evaluation of demineralized bone matrix paste and putty in periodontal intraosseous defects. J Periodontol 2005;76:768–77.

[52] Rabalais ML Jr, Yukna RA, Mayer ET. Evaluation of durapatite ceramic as an alloplastic implant in periodontal osseous defects. I. Initial six-month results. J Periodontol 1981;52:680–9.

[53] Meffert RM, Thomas JR, Hamilton KM, et al. Hydroxylapatite as an alloplastic graft in the treatment of human periodontal osseous defects. J Periodontol 1985;56:63–73.

[54] Yukna RA, Harrison BG, Caudill RF, et al. Evaluation of durapatite ceramic as an alloplastic implant in periodontal osseous defects. II. Twelve month reentry results. J Periodontol 1985;56:540–7.

[55] Mora F, Ouhayoun JP. Clinical evaluation of natural coral and porous hydroxyapatite implants in periodontal bone lesions: results of a 1-year follow-up. J Clin Periodontol 1995;22:877–84.

[56] White E, Shors EC. Biomaterials aspects of Interpore 200 porous hydroxyapatite. Dent Clin North Am 1986;30:49–67.

[57] Yukna RA. Clinical evaluation of coralline calcium carbonate as a bone replacement graft material in human periodontal osseous defects. J Periodontol 1994;65:177–85.

[58] Kim C-K, Choi E-J, Cho K-S, et al. Periodontal repair in intrabony defects treated with a calcium carbonate implant and guided tissue regeneration. J Periodontol 1996;67:1301–6.

[59] Kenney EB, Lekovic V, Han T, et al. The use of a porous hydroxylapatite implant in periodontal defects. I. Clinical results after six months. J Periodontol 1985;56:82–8.

[60] Krejci CB, Bissada NF, Farah C, et al. Clinical evaluation of porous and nonporous hydroxyapatite in the treatment of human periodontal bony defects. J Periodontol 1987;58:521–8.

[61] Kilic AR, Efeoglu E, Yilmaz S. Guided tissue regeneration in conjunction with hydroxyapatite-collagen grafts for infrabony defects: a clinical and radiological evaluation. J Clin Periodontol 1997; 24:372–83.

[62] Okuda K, Tai H, Tanabe K, et al. Platelet-rich plasma combined with a porous hydroxyapatite graft for the treatment of intrabony periodontal defects in humans: a comparative controlled clinical study. J Periodontol 2005;76:890–8.

[63] Yukna RA. HTR polymer grafts in human periodontal osseous defects. I. 6-month clinical results. J Periodontol 1990;61:633–42.

[64] Shahmiri S, Singh IJ, Stahl SS. Clinical response to the use of the HTR polymer implant in human intrabony lesions. Int J Periodontics Restorative Dent 1992;12:294–9.

[65] Hench LL, Wilson J. Surface-active biomaterials. Science 1984;226:630–6.

[66] Froum SJ, Weinberg MA, Tarnow D. Comparison of bioactive glass synthetic bone graft particles and open débridement in the treatment of human periodontal defects: a clinical study. J Periodontol 1998;69:698–709.

[67] Park J-S, Suh J-J, Choi S-H, et al. Effects of pretreatment clinical parameters on bioactive glass implantation in intrabony periodontal defects. J Periodontol 2001;72:730–40.

[68] Ong MM, Eber RM, Korsnes MI, et al. Evaluation of a bioactive glass alloplast in treating periodontal intrabony defects. J Periodontol 1998;69:1346–54.

[69] Bowen JA, Mellonig JT, Gray JL, et al. Comparison of decalcified freeze-dried bone allograft and porous particulate hydroxyapatite in human periodontal osseous defects. J Periodontol 1989;60:647–54.

[70] Baldock WT, Hutchens LH Jr, McFall WT Jr, et al. An evaluation of tricalcium phosphate implants in human periodontal osseous defects of two patients. J Periodontol 1985;56:1–7.

[71] Shepard WK, Bohat O, Joseph CE, et al. Human clinical and histological responses to a calcitite implant in intraosseous lesions. Int J Periodontics Restorative Dent 1986;6(3):46–63.

[72] Stahl SS, Froum S. Histological evaluation of human intraosseous healing responses to the placement of tricalcium phosphate ceramic implants. I. Three to eight months. J Periodontol 1986;57:211–7.

[73] Richardson CR, Mellonig JT, Brunsvold MA, et al. Clinical evaluation of Bio-Oss: a bovine-derived xenograft for the treatment of periodontal osseous defects in humans. J Clin Periodontol 1999;26:421–8.

[74] Paolantonio M. Combined periodontal regenerative technique in human intrabony defects by collagen

membranes and anorganic bovine bone: a controlled clinical study. J Periodontol 2002;73:158–66.

[75] Cortellini P, Tonetti MS. Clinical performance of a regenerative strategy for intrabony defects: scientific evidence and clinical experience. J Periodontol 2005;76:341–50.

[76] Velasquez-Plata D, Scheyer ET, Mellonig JT. Clinical comparison of an enamel matrix derivative used alone or in combination with a bovine-derived xenograft for the treatment of periodontal osseous defects in humans. J Periodontol 2002;73:433–40.

[77] Scheyer ET, Velasquez-Plata D, Brunsvold MA, et al. A clinical comparison of a bovine-derived xenograft used alone or in combination with an enamel matrix derivative for the treatment of periodontal osseous defects in humans. J Periodontol 2002;73:423–32.

[78] Yukna RA, Krauser JT, Callan DP, et al. Multi-center clinical comparison of combination anorganic bovine-derived hydroxyapatite matrix (ABM)/cell binding peptide (P-15) and ABM in human periodontal osseous defects: 6-month results. J Periodontol 2000;71:1671–9.

[79] Hallman M, Lundgren S, Sennerby L. Histologic analysis of clinical biopsies taken 6 months and 3 years after maxillary sinus floor augmentation with 80% bovine hydroxyapatite and 20% autogenous bone mixed with fibrin glue. Clin Implant Dent Relat Res 2001;3:87–96.

[80] Valentini P, Abensur D. Maxillary sinus floor elevation for implant placement with demineralized freeze-dried bone and bovine bone (Bio-Oss): a clinical study of 20 patients. Int J Periodontics Restorative Dent 1997;17:232–41.

[81] Yukna RA, Evans GH, Aichelmann-Reidy MB, et al. Clinical comparison of bioactive glass bone replacement graft material and expanded polytetrafluoroethylene barrier membrane in treating human mandibular molar class II furcations. J Periodontol 2001;72:125–33.

[82] Calongne KB, Aichelmann-Reidy MB, Yukna RA, et al. Clinical comparison of microporous biocompatible composite of PMMA, PHEMA and calcium hydroxide grafts and expanded polytetrafluoroethylene barrier membranes in human mandibular class II furcations: a case series. J Periodontol 2001;72:1451–9.

[83] Lamb JT, Greenwell H, Drisko C, et al. A comparison of porous and non-porous teflon membranes plus demineralized freeze-dried bone allograft in the treatment of class II buccal/lingual furcation defects: a clinical reentry study. J Periodontol 2001;72:1580–7.

[84] Tonetti MS, Prini Prato G, Cortellini P. Effect of cigarette smoking on periodontal healing following GTR in infrabony defects: a preliminary retrospective study. J Clin Periodontol 1995;22:229–34.

[85] Cortellini P, Pini Prato G, Tonetti MS. Periodontal regeneration of human infrabony defects. V. Effect of oral hygiene on long term stability. J Clin Periodontol 1994;21:606–10.

ELSEVIER
SAUNDERS

Oral Maxillofacial Surg Clin N Am 19 (2007) 513–521

**ORAL AND
MAXILLOFACIAL
SURGERY CLINICS
of North America**

A Review of Bone Substitutes

Solon T. Kao, DDS[a,b,*], Daniel D. Scott, DMD[c]

[a]*Oral and Maxillofacial Surgery, Medical College of Georgia School of Dentistry, Augusta, GA, USA*
[b]*Department of Surgery, Medical College of Georgia School of Medicine, Augusta, GA, USA*
[c]*Oral and Maxillofacial Surgery Residency Program, Medical College of Georgia School of Medicine,
Augusta, GA, USA*

Bone grafting techniques have been used by medical specialists for more than 100 years. In the year 1879, Macewen [1] successfully replaced the proximal two thirds of a humerus in a 4-year-old child with allograft bone. Currently, more than 500,000 bone grafting procedures are performed yearly in the United States in the fields of dentistry, neurosurgery, and orthopaedics [2]. There are many applications for using bone and bone substitutes in medicine, including restoring form and function to the skeletal structure, providing stabilization, and enabling aesthetic modifications. The bone-grafting process is not a new procedure in the field of oral and maxillofacial surgery. Surgeons have been performing autologous grafts to the cranial facial region for many years. Increasing popularity of dental implant surgery has created heavy demand for dentoalveolar reconstruction, such as sinus augmentation procedures and immediate implant procedures. This new trend in dentistry for implants has created a surge in new grafting products for the dental and medical community. Options currently include allograft, xenograft, and synthetic grafting materials, with each manufacturer claiming wonderful results (Tables 1 and 2). Prospective grafting materials most likely will be totally synthetic and yield no chance of transmitting diseases. Regardless of the advancements in technology, grafting materials must obey the nature of bone healing. A grafting material must be able to withstand being washed away by the initial hemorrhage/inflammation phase. It also must allow penetration of host vascular tissue and fibrous granulation with subsequent macrophage action, which leads to proper revascularization and induction of osteoclasts and osteoblasts, permitting osseointegration. The topic of bone substitutes is broad in scope. This article presents an overview of bone substitutes.

Overview

Many factors are involved in the successful incorporation of a grafted material, including graft type, preparation site, vascularity, mechanical strength, and pore size of the material. These parameters make the use of bone substitutes challenging in terms of reliability and predictability. Selecting the graft material is based on many factors. One such factor deals with the morbidity of the harvest site, which occurs in autograft harvesting. Another important area to consider is whether the graft primarily provides mechanical or biologic support. The individual features also have an effect on the graft material chosen, the success of the graft, and the overall results of the surgery.

The four desired properties of bone graft materials are osteogenesis, osteoinduction, osteoconduction, and osteointegration. The only graft material that contains all four qualities is autologous bone. For this reason it continues to be the gold standard in bone grafting (Fig. 1). Osteogenesis is new bone formation that occurs from osteoprogenitor cells that are present in the graft, survive the transplant, and proliferate and

---

* Corresponding author. Oral and Maxillofacial Surgery, Medical College of Georgia School of Dentistry, AD 1207, Augusta, GA 30912.
E-mail address: skao@mcg.edu (S.T. Kao).

Table 1
Bone substitute synopsis

Graft material	Characteristics	Examples
Allograft	A graft that is taken from a member of the same species as the host but is genetically dissimilar	Cadaver cortical/ cancellous bone, FDBA, DFDBA
Xenograft	Grafts derived from a genetically different species than the host	Bio-Oss, coralline HA, red algae
Alloplast (synthetic materials)	Fabricated graft materials	Calcium sulfate, bioactive glasses, HA, NiTi

Abbreviations: DFDBA, decalcified freeze-dried bone allograft; FDBA, freeze-dried bone allograft; HA, hydroxyapatite; NiTi, porous nickel titanium.

differentiate to osteoblasts [2]. During autologous grafting, cancellous trabecular structure with osteoblasts makes an attractive area for bone regeneration. Marrow elements provide the fusion bed with osteoinductive proteins, potential osteogenic cells, and a local blood supply, which make osteogenesis possible [3].

The process of osteoinduction entails the stimulation and recruitment of nearby undifferentiated mesenchymal stem cells to the graft site.

Table 2
Bone graft material characteristics

Characteristic	Graft material
Osteogenesis	Autograft
Osteoinduction	BMP
	DFDBA
	DBM
Osteoconduction	Bio-Oss
	Calcium phosphates
	Calcium sulfate
	Collagen
	FDBA
	Glass ionomers
	HA
	NiTi

Abbreviations: BMP, bone morphogenetic protein; DBM, demineralized bone matrix; DFDBA, decalcified freeze-dried bone allograft; FDBA, freeze-dried bone allograft. HA, hydroxyapatite; NiTi, porous nickel titanium.

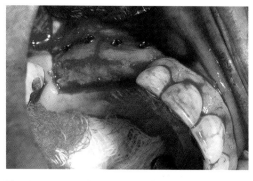

Fig. 1. Four months status post successful autologous graft with allograft at the border.

Once at the graft site, the stem cells are triggered to differentiate into chondrocytes and osteoblasts. The method of recruitment and differentiation occurs through a cascade of events triggered by graft-derived factors called bone morphogenetic proteins (BMP) -2, -4, -7, which are members of the transforming growth factor-β superfamily. These BMPs are present in the matrix of the graft and are accessed after the mineral content of the bone graft has been removed. In addition to the BMPs, a list of other vital factors used in healing includes platelet-derived growth factors, fibroblast growth factors, insulin-like growth factors, granulocyte colony-stimulating factors, mitogens, and interleukins. Angiogenic factors, such as vascular endothelial-derived growth factor, also are present [2,4].

Osteoconduction is the ingrowth of vascular tissue and mesenchymal stem cells into the scaffold structure presented by the graft material. This is an ordered process that results in the formation of new haversian systems in a predictable pattern along the host-graft interface, which subsequently infuse into the graft material [4]. Osteointegration is described as bonding of the host and the graft material [2]. This phenomenon is vital to graft survival. For the graft to be functional, an adequate amount of new bone must exist in the graft and unite with the host bone [4].

Allograft

Although autografts are the gold standard, allografts are much more accepted by patients as the bone grafting material of choice. Allogeneic bone is a graft that is taken from a member of the same species as the host but is genetically dissimilar. Approximately one third of the bone grafts in the United States currently are allografts [2]. The grafts are prepared as fresh, frozen, freeze-dried, mineralized, and demineralized, and each preparation may be purchased as cortical chips, cortical granules, cortical wedges, or cancellous powder. The properties of the allograft are directly related to the steps taken in processing the material. Most allografts are harvested, processed, and distributed through the American Association of Tissue Banks. Because of the strict regulations adopted by the American Association of Tissue Banks, the rate of disease transmission has almost halted. The risk of contracting HIV is estimated to be 1 in 1.6 million, as compared with the risk of 1 in 450,000 in blood transfusions [4]. Rigorous background checks are performed on the donor and his or her family before the donor is accepted into the program.

Once the grafts are harvested, they are processed through different methods, including physical débridement, ultrasonic washing, treatment with ethylene oxide, antibiotic washing, and gamma irradiation for spore elimination. With this additional processing, however, the graft's biologic and mechanical properties are weakened [5]. The goal of these steps is to remove antigenic components and reduce host immune response while retaining the biologic characteristic of the graft [4]. Fresh or frozen allografts possess the highest osteoinductive and osteoconductive potential, but they are rarely used because of increased risk of host immune response and disease transmission. Compared with freeze-dried allografts, fresh or frozen allografts induce much stronger immune response, which is the primary reason why processed grafts are favored [3].

Freeze-dried, or lyophilized, grafts are the least immunogenic, but they possess inferior osteoinductive properties, mechanical properties, and strength compared with fresh or frozen [6]. Host immune response and infection are reduced by eliminating the cellular phase of the allograft. Although freeze drying kills all cells, the chemical integrity of the graft remains intact [7]. Processing freeze-dried demineralized bone involves placing the graft in antibiotic wash twice at 4°C for 1 hour. Then the material is stored at −70°C to dry up to 5% of water. Another favorable finding is that HIV has not been transmitted in freeze-dried bone [8]. Although the graft undergoes lyophilization, microfractures form along the collagen fibers. These cracks result in a decrease in the mechanical properties of the graft. To minimize the effects of these fractures, it is advised to rehydrate the specimen before use to regain some of the lost properties [2,4].

Mineralized grafts contain osteoconductive properties but lack osteoinductive capabilities. Graft incorporation with the host bone is possible by the graft acting as a scaffold that supports bone ingrowth through the structure. Research shows that pore sizes that range from 150 to 500 μm provide optimum opportunity for graft incorporation [9]. The mineral retained in the tissue not only provides framework support but also affects the host cell response. Graft materials, such as freeze-dried bone allograft (FDBA), have proved to be successful in osseous grafting. This material is often used in periodontal regenerative procedures and covered with a membrane. A study by Piattelli and colleagues [10] found that FDBA performed better than its counterpart—demineralized freeze-dried bone allograft (DFDBA). Their research noted osteocytes and haversian systems found in FDBA grafts, whereas the osteocytic lacunae in the DFDBA mostly remained empty. The study also noted that FDBA particles farthest away from the host-graft interface were embedded in new bone, whereas DFDBA particles farthest away from the host-graft interface were surrounded with connective tissue.

When DFDBA was compared with autologous bone in maxillary sinus augmentations, DFDBA showed 29% new bone formation compared with 40% with autologous bone [11]. It was also noted that the DFDBA particles located near pre-existing bone were surrounded by new bone, but the particles located near the center of the graft showed no signs of remineralization or new bone formation [11]. This product has shown positive results in periodontal regenerative surgery and maxillofacial dental implant surgery. From my personal experiences, I have received consistent great results from DFDBA (Fig. 2). I believe that this material has a wide range of application in dentoalveolar grafting procedure at low-stress areas. DFDBA does not necessarily remove all minerals from the graft. I would like to share with the readers about the manufacturing process of DFDBA. In 1965, Marshall Urist described the process of osteoinduction, which was obtained by acid demineralizing the bone before implantation. Acid demineralization is usually done by processing graft in 0.5 to 0.6 molar hydrochloric acid. For adequate osteoinductive properties to be present, at least 40% of the mineral content must be removed [4]. The demineralization

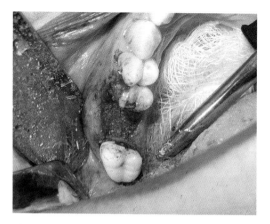

Fig. 2. Immediate placement of allograft placed at extraction site.

process is sensitive. It has been shown that the osteoinductive properties of grafts are removed if the calcium content of the demineralized graft is less than 2% by weight [12]. Through this discovery, researchers noted that providing calcium ions in the graft shows benefit during mineralization [13].

Demineralized bone matrix (DBM) is an option as an allograft material for defect repair. It is produced through decalcification of cortical bone. Because of the processing method, it is found to be more osteoinductive than standard mineralized allograft while retaining most of the bone growth factors after removal of the mineral phase. The advantage to using DBM is its ability to be molded to fill the desired area with graft material. One disadvantage of this material is the technical challenge associated with its low viscosity. Once placed in the defect, some of the material may become displaced and provide no benefit to the grafting procedure. Recently, excipients have been added to the DBM. Excipients are usually inert substances that act as transport vehicles. They are often used in drug preparations. One popular example is poloxamer 407, which is a reverse-phase copolymer that becomes a more viscous gel when warmed to body temperature [14]. Once the DBM and the excipient are combined, the mixture begins to harden at the surgical site, which allows for better handling and adaptability. Another benefit to using this copolymer is the slow release of active ingredients, such as BMPs [14]. Other copolymers are available, such as polyglycolic/poly-L-lactic acid, but they have been shown to resorb slower and leave voids within the healing area, which may result in fibrous tissue healing [9].

The mineral content of the allograft directly affects how additional proteins/factors can be used at the grafting site. Mineralized bone matrix has no osteoinductive properties, and BMPs are encased by the bone minerals [9]. By decreasing mineral content in the graft, the osteoinductive property is elevated by making growth factors more available to stimulate mesenchymal cells. Unfortunately, reduction of mineral content decreases mechanical strength of the graft. Demineralization is a compromise. Studies showed that demineralized implants do not undergo resorption during bone induction, in contrast to mineral-containing powered implants, which are resorbed without bone production [15].

Another type of grafting material available on the market is collagen based (eg, extracellular bone matrix). Collagen contributes to mineral deposition, vascular ingrowth, and growth factor binding, which provides a favorable environment for bone regeneration [12]. Additional features of collagen include its potential for immunogenicity and its diminished structural integrity. Giannoudis and colleagues [2] noted that collagen is a poor graft substitute, but it does significantly increase graft incorporation when combined with BMPs or a carrier such as hydroxyapatite.

Xenograft

Xenografts are derived from a genetically different species than the host. One of the most used xenografts is bovine bone. The best known example of this is Bio-Oss (Osteohealth, Shirley, NY). Bio-Oss, deproteinized bovine bone mineral, has been treated by having all of its organic material removed. This treatment leaves a crystal structure that practically matches human cancellous bone in structure. The particle size of this material is 0.25 to 1 mm. Pores with these dimensions have been shown to promote osteogenesis [16]. Bio-Oss has 75% of its volume contained in its porous scaffold. This structure greatly increases the surface area and results in a material that is good for osteoconduction, but because of its large porous nature, the initial stability may be compromised [17]. This large surface area increases angiogenesis and enhances new bone growth [18]. In a study that compared Bio-Oss to autologous bone in maxillary sinus augmentation procedures, Bio-Oss resulted in 39% new bone formation compared with 40% with autologous bone after 6 months [11]. These results showed the effectiveness of this substitute material by almost matching the amount of new bone formation as seen with autologous bone. Although the results of new bone generation were nearly similar at 6 months, 31% of the grafted Bio-Oss was still present at the graft site as compared with only 18% with autologous bone [11]. It is still unknown whether this substitute completely resorbs. In 1992, Klinge and colleagues [19], noted total resorption of Bio-Oss granules at 14 weeks after placement in rabbit skulls. Skoglund and colleagues [20] reported that granules were present even after 44 months. Although all the aspects of this material have not shown similar results, this material has proved to be a workhorse in oral surgery.

Another popular alternative xenograft is coralline hydroxyapatite, which is made from ocean coral. Coralline hydroxyapatite, marketed as ProOsteon (Interpore International, Irvine, CA), has been available since the 1970s. This material was created with the intention of producing a graft material with a more consistent pore size. Coral, which is composed mostly of calcium carbonate, is processed to remove most of the organic content. Then it is subjected to high pressure and heat in the presence of an aqueous phosphate solution. When the process is complete, the calcium carbonate coral skeleton is totally replaced with a calcium phosphate skeleton. The material is sterilized in this process concurrently [21]. Hulbert and colleagues [22] found that a pore size of 45 to 100 μm is required for bone ingrowth into ceramic materials. They also noted that pore sizes of 100 to 150 μm allow for faster ingrowth of fibrovascular tissues. Researchers have found that nanoparticular hydroxyapatite not only provides the benefits of traditional hydroxyapatites but also resorbs. The material provides only minimal dimensional stability, but when combined with 25% autogenous bone, the dimensional stability was found to be sufficient [23].

Other xenografts that are being studied by researchers include chitosan, gusuibu, and red algae [24–26]. Chitosan is a product of the exoskeleton of crustaceans, and it shows the ability to stimulate mesenchymal stem cells to differentiate into osteoblasts. When this product is combined with hydroxyapatite, the osteoconductive potential of the graft is increased [24]. Gusuibu is a rhizome of the perennial pteridophyte *Drynaria fortunei*. This herb shows osteoinductive capabilities and increased alkaline phosphatase activity and has a positive effect on promoting calcification [26]. Another potentially useful xenograft material comes from red algae. Researchers have the ability to chemically convert red algae to hydroxyapatite, which is then used in grafting defects [25].

Synthetic materials

Synthetic grafting materials have been shown to possess two of the four characteristics of an ideal graft: osteoconduction and osteointegration. The ideal synthetic graft material should be biocompatible and elicit minimal fibrotic changes. The graft should support new bone growth and undergo remodeling. Other features include similar toughness, modulus of elasticity, and compressive strength compared with host cortical or cancellous bone [21]. Many synthetic materials are available to surgeons, including bioactive glasses, glass ionomers, aluminum oxide, calcium sulfate, calcium phosphates, α- and β-tricalcium phosphate (TCP), and synthetic hydroxyapatite [21].

The bioactive glasses are nonporous and consist of silicon dioxide (SiO_2), calcium oxide (CaO), phosphorus pentoxide (P_2O_5), and sodium oxide (Na_2O). Solubility is directly related to the proportion of sodium oxide found in the formulation. By altering the concentrations of sodium oxide, silicon dioxide, and calcium oxide, glasses with different properties are produced [27]. These materials exhibit significantly greater strength compared with calcium phosphates. A positive feature with the use of these substitutes includes the formation of a strong bond between the glass and the host bone, which is accomplished through hydroxyapatite crystals [28].

Glass ionomers are porous, which leads to bone ingrowth through their osteoconductive nature. One possible advantage to using this product is its ability to be impregnated with antibiotics for slow release. One disadvantage with the use of this product is that it does not resorb [21]. Glass ionomers have been considered as replacements for polymethylmethacrylate bone cement, which generates significant heat during polymerization [29]. Glass ionomers possess a working time of approximately 5 minutes. After 24 hours, they possess a modulus of elasticity and compressive strength that is similar to cortical bone [30,31]. Glass ionomers have been used to seal defects in the skull, but care must be taken not to let them come into contact with cerebrospinal fluid or neural tissue. These precautions are taken because aluminium ions and polyacid in its unset form are neurotoxic [32]. Other than its uses in dentistry, glass ionomers have been used by otorhinolaryngologic surgeons for auditory ossicular reconstructions and sinus augmentations [21].

Aluminum oxide is found as a component of multiple bioactive materials, but this material also can be used by itself as a graft material. One feature of this type of graft is that the chemical does not exchange ions with the host; therefore, there is no osteointegration. Aluminum oxides are rigid and have been used as graft expanders [21]. Uses of this substitute include orbital implants, ossicular replacements, and prosthetic joint linings [33].

Calcium sulfate ($CaSO_4 \cdot \frac{1}{2} H_2O$), also known as plaster of Paris, has been used for more than a century. In 1892, Trendelenburg's clinic in Bonn reported the use of a mixture of plaster of Paris with a 5% solution of phenol in the treatment of defects in various bones in eight patients [34]. After this initial trial, calcium sulfate was not reported to be used again until 1925. Since then, it steadily grew in popularity and use for many years. Key features of this alloplast material include its biocompatibility, rapid resorption rate, and unique ability to stimulate osteogenesis [35]. An additional use for calcium sulfate is its reported use as a binding and stabilizing agent [36]. The matrix is osteoconductive, which leads to new vessel ingrowth and fibrous and osseous ingrowth. One critical feature is that the material must be near viable periosteum or endosteum. After the graft is placed, it is resorbed over the next 7 weeks through dissolution [37]. In 1981, Beeson [38] noted that calcium sulfate is normally resorbed concurrently with deposition of new autogenous cancellous bone.

Calcium phosphates do not possess osteogenic or osteoinductive properties. They use their osteointegrative property by the formation of hydroxyapatite on the surface after the graft is placed [39]. These materials have a good history of biocompatibility with no reported foreign body reactions [40]. Examples of calcium phosphates include α- and β-TCP and hydroxyapatite. α-TCP is available in an injectable form (Norian-SRS) combined with calcium carbonate and monocalcium phosphate monohydrate. This mixture is prepared and injected into the defect, at which time it hardens with minimal thermal generation. Once hardened, this material yields a maximum compressive strength of approximately 55 MPa, which is similar to the compressive strength of human cancellous bone [41]. Although the compressive strengths are comparable, this material yields a tensile strength that is much lower than that of human cancellous bone [42]. This product undergoes long-term remodeling, and the graft is eventually replaced through new bone formation. Research shows that this material initially displays osteointegration, which is succeeded by incorporation [2].

An important aspect about α-TCP in the form of calcium phosphate cements is that it is technique sensitive. If the material does not set in the defect before the incision is closed, it may become contaminated by fluid. Postoperatively, the unset material dissociates into small particles, which leads to giant cell–related inflammatory reactions [9]. A study by Kurashina and colleagues [43] showed that unset α-TCP had flown away from the grafting site and failed to set in the presence of blood. Pioletti and colleagues [44] confirmed additional findings that showed that small particulate-sized calcium phosphate cements are phagocytized by macrophages and multinucleated giant cells. This process results in the accumulation of calcium in the mitochondria and eventually leads to lysis and cell death. These findings concerning the potential disadvantages of α-TCP–related calcium phosphate cements cannot be ignored.

β-TCPs have been in use for many years. Many features of this material make its use appealing. β-TCP shows great osteoconductive potential because of its macroporosity (ranging from 1–1000 μm), which leads to good bone ingrowth [45]. Approximately 90% of this material is interconnected void spaces [2]. β-TCP also bonds directly to bone, which facilitates healing [46]. The healing of a β-TCP graft occurs in multiple phases. The first phase results in absorption of the host bone, which is followed by new bone apposition on the graft material. The next phase includes absorption of the graft material, with remodeling taking place. Another feature of β-TCP is that no macrophages or giant cells are found during the healing process [45]. Recent studies have focused on creating biphasic TCPs composed of alpha and beta forms of TCP. The combination of the two phases of TCP yields a material that is more biodegradable that β-TCP alone [47].

Synthetic hydroxyapatite, $C_{10}(PO_4)_6(OH)_2$, has been available for more than 30 years. It is the primary mineral found in bone. Synthetic hydroxyapatite can be found as porous or nonporous and in ceramic or nonceramic forms. The ceramic forms are virtually nonresorbable, occurring at a rate of 1% to 2% per year [33]. In block form, synthetic hydroxyapatite is hard to shape, and it does not allow fibro-osseous ingrowth [21]. These materials have been used to coat implants because of their great osteointegrative capabilities [48,49].

Composite grafts have developed a history of use over the last few decades as a material for use in repair of open alveolar clefts. Composite grafts are composed of autogenous corticocancellous bone mixed with hydroxyapatite, collagen, blood, and bacitracin powder [34]. Although this material has a history of high success, it is often overlooked by surgeons because of the development of newer products. Nickel-titanium is currently being studied as a material used in grafting because of its good strength and elastic modulus properties. Under nonloading conditions, good bone ingrowth can result using nickel-titanium with pore sizes of 50 to 125 μm [50]. Another feature that is required for bone ingrowth using metal implants is the need for interconnecting fenestrations that provide spacing for vascular tissue, which, in turn, allows for continued mineralization of the bone [51,52].

Another synthetic material available is PepGen P-15 (Dentsply Friadent CeraMed, Lakewood, CO). PepGen P-15 is a peptide that is 15 amino acids in length. It is identical to the 15 amino acid sequence between 766 and 780 amino acids of type 1 collagen's α-1 chain [53,54]. This peptide is then combined with anorganic bovine bone to yield a successful substitute with a multifocal approach to bone healing. The mineral content present in the bovine bone provides a structure that is highly osteoconductive [11]. The P-15 is available to attach to cell surface sites on collagen. This binding stabilizes the cells and promotes differentiation [55]. Scarano and colleagues [11], found that P-15 yielded 37% new bone formation at grafted maxillary sinus augmentation sites compared with 40% new bone formation with grafted autologous bone. Researchers have yet to develop a material that outperforms autologous bone, but PepGen P-15 shows promising results as a substitute.

In addition to these materials, research is continuing to modify the products with hopes of creating a graft that incorporates faster, resorbs, and yields a bony union that resembles natural form and structure.

Summary

The allograft is the most popular graft used currently. This graft type can be purchased in multiple structures depending on the clinical need for defect repair. Synthetic substitutes create a new avenue for clinicians to explore as adjuncts in surgical procedures. These materials may not necessarily be used solely for reconstructive procedures, but when used in the right situations in combination with autologous, allograft, or other synthetics, the results have the potential for more desirable results. The future of bone graft substitutes will continue to expand with increasing technologic advances, which allow us to better understand bone healing, the role that factors such as BMP, transforming growth factor, platelet-derived growth factor, and others play in this process, and how to better induce these processes when desired. Researchers are steadily understanding materials better and learning how to manipulate those materials and harness the desired properties while removing the undesired properties to create ideal graft substitutes.

When bony reconstruction is presented to the surgeon, many choices must be weighed before the proper graft material is chosen. The site of reconstruction, size of the defect to repair, objectives of the surgery, examination of the patient, desires of the patient, and knowledge of graft materials are all factors that must be entertained before the surgery begins. There are many options in graft materials from which to choose, all with advantages and disadvantages. Knowledge of this information distinguishes a good surgeon from a great surgeon.

References

[1] Macewen W. Observation concerning transplantation of bone: illustrated by a case of interhuman osseous transplantation whereby over two thirds of the shaft of a humerus was restored. Proceedings of the Royal Society of London 1881;32:232–47.

[2] Giannoudis PV, Dinopoulos H, Tsiridis E. Bone substitutes: an update. Injury, International Journal of the Care of the Injured 2005;36S:S20–7.

[3] Strong DM, Friedlanender GE, Tomford WW, et al. Immunologic responses in human recipients of osseous and osteochondral allografts. Clin Orthop 1996; 326:107–14.

[4] Khan SN, Cammisa FP Jr, Sandhy HS, et al. The biology of bone grafting. J Am Acad Orthop Surg 2005;13(1):77–86.

[5] Ehrler DM, Vaccaro AR. The use of allograft bone in lumbar spine surgery. Clin Orthop 2000;371: 38–45.

[6] Gazdag AR, Lane JM, Glaser D, et al. Alternative to autogenous bone graft: efficacy and indications. J Am Acad Orthop Surg 1995;3:1–8.

[7] Mellonig JT. Autogenous and allogeneic bone grafts in periodontal therapy. Crit Rev Oral Biol Med 1991;3(4):333–52.

[8] Cornell CN. Osteoconductive materials and their role as substitutes for autogenous bone grafts. Orthop Clin North Am 1999;30:591–8.

[9] Moghadam HG, Sándor GKB, Holmes HHI, et al. Histomorphometric evaluation of bone regeneration using allogeneic and alloplastic bone substitutes. J Oral Maxillofac Surg 2004;62:202–13.

[10] Piattelli A, Scarano A, Corgliano M, et al. Comparison of bone regeneration with the use of mineralized and demineralized freeze-dried bone allografts: a histological and histochemical study in man. Biomaterials 1996;17:1127–31.

[11] Scarano A, Degidi M, Iezzi G, et al. Maxillary sinus augmentation with different biomaterials: a comparative histologic and histomorphometric study in man. Implant Dent 2006;15(2):197–207.

[12] Zhang M, Powers RM, Wolfinbarger L Jr. Effect(s) of the demineralization process on the osteoinductivity of demineralized bone matrix. J Periodontol 1997;68:1085–92.

[13] Murakami T, Murakami H, Ramp WK, et al. Calcium hydroxide ameliorates tobramycin toxicity in cultured chick tibiae. Bone 1997;21:411–8.

[14] Coulson R, Clokie CM, Peel S. Collagen and thermally reversible poloxamer deliver demineralized bone matrix and biologically active proteins to site of bone regeneration. Presented at the Portland Bone Symposium. Portland (OR): 1999. p. 619–27.

[15] Glowacki J, Altobelli D, Mulliken JB. The fate of mineralized and demineralized osseous implants in cranial defects. Calcif Tissue Int 1981;33:71–6.

[16] Misch CE. Contemporary implant dentistry: bone augmentation for implant placement: keys to bone grafting. 2nd edition. St. Louis (MO): Mosby; 1998. p. 451–67.

[17] Su-Gwan K, Hak-Kyun K, Sung-Chul L. Combined implantation of particulate dentine, plaster of Paris, and a bone xenograft (Bio-Oss) for bone regeneration in rats. J Craniomaxillofac Surg 2001; 29:282–8.

[18] Rodriguez A, Anastassov GE, Lee H, et al. Maxillary sinus augmentation with deproteinated bovine bone and platelet rich plasma with simultaneous insertion of endosseous implants. J Oral Maxillofac surg 2003;61:157–63.

[19] Klinge B, Alberius P, Isaksson S, et al. Osseous response to implanted natural bone mineral and synthetic hydroxyapatite ceramic in the repair of experimental skull bone defects. J Oral Maxillofac Surg 1992;50:241–9.

[20] Skoglund A, Hising P, Young C. A clinical and histologic examination in humans of the osseous response to implanted natural bone mineral. Int J Oral Maxillofac Implants 1997;12:194–9.

[21] Moore WR, Graves SE, Bain GI. Synthetic bone graft substitutes. ANZ J Surg 2001;71:354–61.

[22] Hulbert SF, Morrison SJ, Klawitter JJ. Tissue reaction to three ceramics of porous and non porous structures. J Biomed Mater Res 1972;6:347–74.

[23] Thorwarth M, Schultze-Mosgau S, Kessler P, et al. Bone regeneration in osseous defects using a resorbable nanoparticular hydroxyapatite. J Oral Maxillofac Surg 2005;63:1626–33.

[24] Cho BC, Chung HY, Lee DG, et al. The effect of chitosan bead encapsulating calcium sulfate as an injectable bone substitute on consolidation in the mandibular distraction osteogenesis of a dog model. J Oral Maxillofac Surg 2005;63:1753–64.

[25] Ewers R. Maxilla sinus grafting with marine algae derived bone forming material: a clinical report of long-term results. J Oral Maxillofac Surg 2005;63: 1712–23.

[26] Wong RWK, Rabie ABM. Effect of gusuibu graft on bone formation. J Oral Maxillofac Surg 2006;64: 770–7.

[27] Hench LL, Wilson J. Surface active biomaterials. Science 1984;226:630–6.

[28] Gross V, Grandes J. The ultrastructure of the interface between a glass ceramic and bone. J Biomed Mater Res 1981;15:291–305.

[29] Jonck LM, Grobbelaar CJ. The biological compatibility of glass ionomer cement in joint replacement. Clin Mater 1989;4:85–107.

[30] Billington RW, Williams JA. Increase in compressive strength of glass ionomer restorative materials with respect to time. J Oral Rehabil 1991;18:163–8.

[31] Jonck LM, Grobbelaar CJ. Biological evaluation of glass ionomer cement as an interface in total joint replacement. Clin Mater 1989;4:201–24.

[32] Brook IM, Hatton PV. Glass ionomers: bioactive implant materials. Biomaterials 1998;19:565–71.

[33] Constantino PD, Freidman CD. Synthetic bone graft substitutes. Otolaryngol Clin North Am 1994; 27:1037–73.

[34] Habal MB, Reddi AH. Bone grafts and bone substitutes. Philadelphia: W.B. Saunders Company; 1992. p. 243–4, 247.

[35] McKee JC, Bailey BJ. Calcium sulphate as a mandibular implant. Otolaryngol Head Neck Surg 1984;92: 277–86.

[36] Snyders RV, Eppley BL, Krukowsky M. Enhancement of repair in experimental calvarial bone defects using calcium sulphate and dextran beads. J Oral Maxillofac Surg 1993;51:517–24.

[37] Bell WH. Resorption rates of bone and bone substitutes. Oral Surgery 1964;17:650–7.

[38] Beeson WH. Plaster of paris as an alloplastic implant in the frontal sinus. Arch Otolaryngol 1981; 107:664–9.

[39] Blom AW, Cunningham JL, Hughes G, et al. The compatibility of ceramic graft substitutes as allograft extenders for use in impaction grafting of the femur. J Bone Joint Surg Br 2005;87-B:421–5.

[40] Hollinger JO, Batistone GC. Biodegradable bone repair materials. Clin Orthop 1986;207:290–305.

[41] Finkemeier CG. Bone-grafting and bone-graft substitutes. J Bone Joint Surg Am 2002;84-A(3):454–64.

[42] Larsson S. Injectable phosphate cements: a review. Available at: http://www.strykertrauma.org/physicians/usa/wp_hydroset_technical_review_larsson.pdf. Accessed October 1, 2007.

[43] Kurashina K, Kurita H, Kotani A, et al. Experimental cranioplasty and skeletal augmentation using an alpha tricalcium phosphate/dicalcium phosphate dibasic/tetracalcium phosphate monoxide cement: a preliminary short term experiment in rabbits. Biomaterials 1998;19:701–6.

[44] Pioletti DP, Takei H, Lin T, et al. The effects of calcium phosphate cement particles on osteoblasts function. Biomaterials 2000;21:1103–14.

[45] Gaasbeek RDA, Toonen HG, van Heerwaarden RJ, et al. Mechanism of bone incorporation of B-TCP bone substitute in open wedge tibial osteotomy in patients. Biomaterials 2005;26:6713–9.

[46] Kokubo T. Design of bioactive bone substitutes based on biomineralization process. Materials Science and Engineering C 2005;25:97–104.

[47] Li Y, Weng W, Tam KC. Novel highly biodegradable biphasic tricalcium phosphates composed of alpha-tricalcium phosphate and beta-tricalcium phosphate. Acta Biomater 2007;3:251–4.

[48] Bellemans J. Osseointegration in porous coated knee arthroplasty: the influence of component coating type in sheep. Acta Orthop Scand Suppl 1999;288:1–35.

[49] Strnad Z, Strnad J, Povysil C, et al. Effect of plasma sprayed hydroxyapatite coating on the osteoconductivity of commercially pure titanium implants. Int J Oral Maxillofac Implants 2000;15:483–90.

[50] Itälä AI, Ylänen HO, Ekholm C, et al. Pore diameter of more than 100 micron is not requisite for bone ingrowth in rabbits. J Biomed Mater Res 2001;58:679–83.

[51] Hulbert SF, Young FA, Mathews RS, et al. Potential of ceramic materials as permanently implantable skeletal prostheses. J Biomed Mater Res 1970;4:433–56.

[52] van Eeden SP, Ripamonti U. Bone differentiation in porous hydroxyapatite in baboons is regulated by the geometry of the substratum: implications for reconstructive craniofacial surgery. Plast Reconstr Surg 1994;93:959–66.

[53] Bhatnagar RS, Qian JJ, Gough CA. The role in cell binding of beta-blend within helical region in collagen alpha1 (I) chain: structural and biological evidence for conformational tautomerism on fiber surface. J Biomol Struct Dyn 1997;14:547–60.

[54] Qian JJ, Bhatnagar RS. Enhanced cell attachment to anorganic bone mineral in the presence of a synthetic peptide related to collagen. J Biomed Mater Res 1996;31:545–54.

[55] Bhatnagar RS, Qian JJ, Wedrychowska A, et al. Design of biomimetic habitat for tissue engineering with P-15, a synthetic peptide analogue of collagen. Tissue Eng 1999;5:53–65.

ELSEVIER
SAUNDERS

Oral Maxillofacial Surg Clin N Am 19 (2007) 523–534

ORAL AND
MAXILLOFACIAL
SURGERY CLINICS
of North America

Contemporary Concepts in the Treatment of Chronic Osteomyelitis

Vincent Coviello, DDS[a],*, Mark R. Stevens, DDS[b]

[a]*Private Practice, 1510 Grove Ridge #202, Germantown, TN 38138, USA*
[b]*Oral and Maxillofacial Surgery, The Medical College of Georgia, Augusta, GA, USA*

The diagnosis and treatment of chronic osteomyelitis remain oddly enigmatic. Despite relatively standard surgical approaches and a wide variety of antibiotic choices, the clinical course often leads to significant morbidity and much consternation on the part of the practitioner and patient. The Cierny-Mader staging system hints at the complexities of the disease [1]. It is based on anatomic location, physiologic status of patient, and local or systemic factors that affect the immune system, vascularity, or metabolism. It is estimated that up to 30% of osteomyelitis infections become chronic [2]. One problem is the nature of the disease: a low-grade, indolent course with variable degrees of pain, necrosis, osteosclerosis, and suppuration. Treatment courses can become remarkably expensive and require long hospital stays and prolonged antibiotic administration. The general purpose of this article is to survey the new directions in oral surgery, orthopedics, infectious disease, immunology, and radiology that may have application to the treatment of maxillofacial osteomyelitis.

Although the incidence of osteomyelitis has declined precipitously over the years, there are several reasons to believe that practitioners may face new, broad challenges [3]. Consider the basic etiologic patterns of the Waldvogel classifications—(1) hematogenous osteomyelitis, (2) osteomyelitis secondary to a contiguous focus, and (3) chronic osteomyelitis [4]—and it is not difficult to foresee change. Hematogenous spread, although most common in pediatric patients, also preys on the ever-increasing numbers of immunocompromised or debilitated patients in intensive care units. The contiguous focus cohort has evolved from one premised on trauma-related causes to the increasing incidence of failed dental implants and bone grafts (Figs. 1–4). Many cases progress to chronic forms because of the emergence of resistant micro-organisms.

Etiologic considerations

Molecular biology

In the past, much attention was directed toward medical and surgical approaches, yet little progress has been made on establishing more than the rudiments of molecular/cellular pathogenesis. Neutrophils are known to be potent mediators of not only early phagocytosis but also secondary tissue injury through degranulation and oxidants. This effect is normally limited by ingress of macrophages that scavenge dead PMNs and cytokines (eg, tumor necrosis factor-alpha) that induce PMN apoptosis. Recent evidence suggested an inverse relationship between interleukin-6 levels and neutrophil apoptosis, which could lead to a prolonged tissue destruction phase [5]. This mechanism, which has been associated with various proinflammatory diseases, has been implicated in progression to chronic osteomyelitis. Cytokine production also can vary with certain antibiotics commonly used to treat infection, another reminder that the interplay among cell-signaling mediators has a direct influence on treatment modalities [6].

Microbiology

Many issues that relate to infecting organisms are pertinent to contemporary treatment of

* Corresponding author.
 E-mail address: vfcoviello@mac.com (V. Coviello).

1042-3699/07/$ - see front matter © 2007 Elsevier Inc. All rights reserved.
doi:10.1016/j.coms.2007.07.001

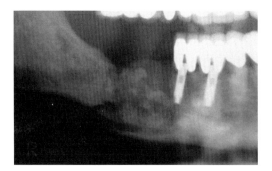

Fig. 1. Implants violate the mucosal barrier and can lead to significant morbidity when infection is not aggressively treated. These implants were originally splinted to two natural teeth, which were removed. Leaving the implants led to progressive bony destruction.

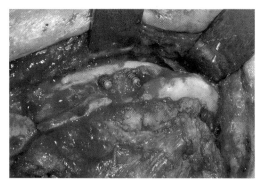

Fig. 3. Intraoperative view of the destruction of medullary and cortical bone secondary to dental implants.

osteomyelitis. One is the emergence of more accurate culturing techniques, which has changed our understanding of the polymicrobial nature of chronic osteomyelitis [7]. Ninety-three percent of osteomyelitic infections of the jaws are polymicrobial, with an average of 3.9 organisms per specimen [8]. Another is the outright change in the identity of the offending microbes. The reality of multidrug resistance has contributed to longer treatment times, increased morbidity, and death. Bacterial tolerance to antibiotics is poorly understood and often negatively affects treatment outcomes [9].

Sound principles in culturing can lead to better clinical outcomes. Cultures should consist of tissue specimens rather than swabs of purulence. The tissue has higher bacterial counts, whereas exuded fluids yield mostly dead organisms and

cellular debris [10]. Specimens should be sent immediately to the microbiology laboratory. Anaerobic species are lost in as little as 15 minutes; aerobes are lost within 2 hours [7]. Proper anaerobic handling takes into account ideal temperatures (37°C) and differing carbon dioxide requirements [11]. Qualitative sensitivity testing is essential and is commonly accomplished through the disk diffusion method. Quantitative sensitivity data may be gathered by serial dilution techniques, which yield the least concentration of antibiotic necessary to inhibit (mean inhibitory concentration) or kill (mean bacterial concentration) the targeted organism [9]. An interesting attempt to bypass bone culture altogether by using blood cultures proved fruitless. Concordance rates between bone and blood samples in 100 patients with osteomyelitis were only 30% [12].

A wide range of organisms contributes to chronic osteomyelitis, and multiple studies have chronicled culture results [8,13,14]. Unlike long

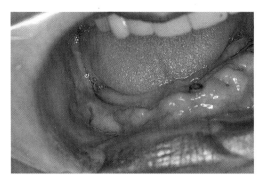

Fig. 2. In this case, some implants were removed, yet the infection persisted. This development validated a diagnosis of osteomyelitis, in which the medullary cavity was seeded directly. This indolent infection led to a mucosal dehiscence that exposed the underlying devitalized bone.

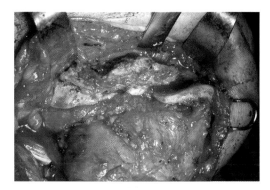

Fig. 4. Similar case of chronic mandibular osteomyelitis resulting from dental implants. Note the large bony sequestrum.

bone osteomyelitis, in which staphylococcal species predominate, the jaws are afflicted with a wide variety of pathogens [15], the most common of which are *Streptococcus, Bacteroides, Lactobacillus, Eubacterium, and Klebsiella* [8]. Even without immunodeficiency, primary mycobacterial and actinomycotic osteomyelitis is a clinical reality [16,17]. Many bacterium that are commonly multidrug resistant, such as *Staphylococcus aureus, Acinetobacter* sp, and *Pseudomonas aeruginosa*, contribute to significant morbidity.

Elucidating the cell biology of drug resistance is critical in the fight against pathogenic organisms. The major mechanisms are beta-lactamases, porin membrane proteins, aminoglycoside-modifying enzymes, topoisomerase mutations, efflux pumps, mobile genetic elements, integrons and polymyxin-specific membrane changes [18]. For *Acinetobacter baumanni*, numerous isolates that contain beta-lactamases, cephalosporinases, and carbapenemases have been found. A troubling emergence of methicillin-resistant *S aureus* with reduced vancomycin susceptibility has been found. In an Australian study that detailed 25 cases, 6 patients suffered from osteomyelitis and all failed vancomycin/glycopeptide courses [19]. *P aeruginosa*, the notorious gram-negative cause of hospital-acquired infection, is often treated with imipenem. Although many strains of carbapenem-resistant *P aeruginosa* have been isolated, the most common mechanism of resistance is an outer membrane protein change [20]. Porins mediate membrane transport, and outer membrane protein structural mutations lead to less antibiotic in the periplasmic space available to bind to receptors [18]. Only polymyxins are effective for panresistant organisms that use various mechanisms synchronously [21].

Host factors

Local and systemic host factors are key in understanding the pathogenesis of osteomyelitis. It has been generally theorized that compromise of local blood flow is a critical factor in predisposition and prolongation of chronic osteomyelitis [22,23]. Laser Doppler flowmetry has been used to confirm that long-standing medullary inflammation leads to appreciable decreases in mandibular blood flow [22]. A critical local factor is violation of standard mucosal or skin barriers with prostheses and grafts. The fundamental first step leading to medullary infection is bacterial seeding of bone and colonization via adhesion or permanent attachment [24]. The subject of slime layer formation and failure of prosthetic implants has been studied extensively in the orthopedic literature. Dental implant placement is an obvious potential source of problems (Fig. 5). Mucosal barrier function often can be subject to breakdown, and peri-implant tissues can be seeded by natural oral flora [25].

Systemic disease can be an important factor in host susceptibility and prolongation of disease. The increased incidence of type 2 diabetes mellitus is dramatic, with 6.2% of Americans currently afflicted [26]. Posttransplant patients are more numerous every day and are afflicted with various organisms, such as *Aspergillus* sp and herpes zoster. Hematogenous seeded osteomyelitis in sickle cell anemia patients is often caused by *Salmonella* or *Klebsiella* spp [27]. Chronic debilitated patients in intensive care units or anyone with long-term indwelling catheters may develop *Pseudomonas* sp osteomyelitis. Intravenous drug abusers are often victims of blood-borne osteomyelitis, usually involving *Serratia* sp, *S aureus, Staphylococcus epidermidis*, or *P aeruginosa*.

Diagnostic components

Part of the continuing concern in diagnosis of chronic osteomyelitis is the sensitivity necessary to detect (1) initiation of disease, (2) the transition from an acute condition, (3) a low-grade clinical entity, and (4) surveillance, especially after surgical intervention or where a local implant exists. The components have not changed over time and consist of patient description, clinical course, practitioner judgment, bone cultures, and imaging. Of these, most advances have been in imaging modalities, which constitutes the bulk of the

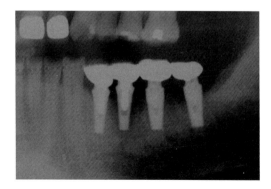

Fig. 5. A subtle radiographic depiction of chronic osteomyelitis in which the damage has been limited to the intramedullary space.

summary in this section. A more subtle change
should be occurring in the index of suspicion that
practitioners carry when considering specific, well-
characterized situations. For instance, a patient
who has uncontrolled diabetes and recalcitrant
sinus disease, ocular acuity/mobility changes, and
subtle (if any) CT changes should be screened for
fungal disease.

Imaging

Conventional radiographs

These techniques are reserved for initial screening purposes for various reasons. For early disease
confined to the marrow spaces, there is a late
change in plain radiographs. It has been estimated
that a 30% reduction in mineralized bone density
must be realized before radiographic changes are
seen. The full implications of osteomyelitic bone
dissolution are not seen for 3 weeks [22,28–30],
which roughly correlates to the first manifestations of reactive bone deposition that follows the
initial destruction of the anorganic matrix [28].
Eventual cortical changes can manifest as osteoly-
sis but sometimes as periosteal/endosteal remodeling, cortical thickening, and sclerosis. A greater
degree of uncertainty exists posttraumatically
with implants and prior bone grafts and where
débridement has been performed. Reported sensitivity and specificity rates for plain films are 14%
and 70%, respectively [31]. These rates limit plain
film use to initial support of clinical suspicion and
added information for the selection and interpre-
tation of further imaging modalities.

CT

Recent advances in CT technology, such as
thin-slice multiplanar reconstructions and helical
imaging, have increased overall use in the diagnosis
of chronic osteomyelitis. There is an obvious
advantage to using CT when assessing bony
destruction, endosteal/periosteal activity, and
medullary sequestra (Fig. 6). Many problems are
encountered with detection of active, low-grade
degradation of bone, however, as is distortion
when hardware is present. Overall, soft tissue contrast resolution is inferior to that of MRI for delin-
eation of abscess cavities or fistulae [32]. The role of
CT scans has expanded to include combination
with single-photon emission CT. Using this type
of imaging, the quantitative image analysis of active low-grade disease offered by scintigraphy can
be defined anatomically by CT [33]. Currently,

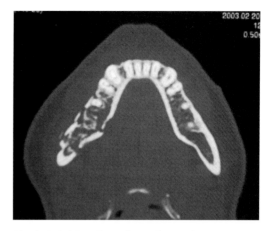

Fig. 6. Axial CT of an advanced case of chronic osteomyelitis depicts obvious cortical destruction. This study
was useful in initial delimiting of resection margins.

CT scanning as a single modality may be useful in
the initial surgical treatment planning for patients
with overt bony destruction. A recent systematic
meta-analysis of orthopedic literature does not
regard CT as a front-line imaging modality for
the assessment of chronic osteomyelitis [33].

MRI

Because of the ability to detect active changes
in bone marrow and surrounding soft tissues,
MRI has been recognized as useful in detecting
acute and early osteomyelitis. In early disease, fat-
suppressed T2 images identify bone marrow
edema, and extracortical soft tissue involvement
is clearly demarcated. There is the added benefit
of no radiation exposure to the patient. High
sensitivities and accurate spatial resolutions also
are apparent in characterizing the bone alterations
of chronic osteomyelitis. T1-weighted, contrast-
enhanced images clearly depict bone marrow
heterogeneity in low-grade, indolent cases. In
posttraumatic and postsurgical patients, T2-
weighted images after intravenous gadolinium
are relatively nonspecific [34,35], which is caused
by hyperemia and enhanced endothelial perme-
ability that often leads to equivocal results. Re-
parative fibrovascular scarring in bone marrow
and soft tissue may hinder specificity for up to
12 months after surgical intervention [32].

To put it simply, MRI has limited ability to
discriminate between edema and outright infection. The presence of metal implants renders MRI
of little diagnostic value. Numerous studies have
documented MRI specificity and sensitivity,

which average 85% and 60%, respectively [34]. A prospective study limited to mandibular osteomyelitis concluded no difference in sensitivity between MRI and scintigraphy [28]. Gadolinium-enhanced MRI offers a sensitive tool in the early presurgical diagnosis of chronic osteomyelitis, although surveillance may be best accomplished with a nuclear medicine technique.

Nuclear medicine

Modern nuclear scans are based on the imaging device and the radiolabeled tracers that target one of the consecutive steps of the host response to infection. A review of scanners is beyond the scope of this article, but they break down categorically into gamma cameras and positron emission tomography scanners. For chronic osteomyelitis, some of the available radiopharmaceuticals (and techniques) include (1) [99mTc] nanocolloid, (2) in vitro labeling with [111In] or [99m Tc] of autologous leukocytes, (3) in vivo labeling of granulocytes with antibodies/[99mTc], (4) gallium-citrate [36], and (5) fluorine-18

fluorodeoxyglucose [32]. Recent systematic meta-analysis of the orthopedic literature showed that fluorodeoxyglucose-positron emission tomography is the most sensitive technique for detecting chronic osteomyelitis, with greater specificity than MRI or leukocyte or bone scintigraphy [34]. This method takes into account the fact that activated neutrophils and macrophages of inflammatory reactions have increased glucose uptake [37,38]. False-negative findings have been documented in tumor patients with elevated blood glucose, yet this does not seem to affect the sensitivity of studies for infectious disease [39].

Problems with resolution have been addressed by effectively combining the study with CT maps (Fig. 7). Because of the high cost and limited availability, this modality has not yet been integrated as a primary diagnosis and surveillance tool [38]. The gold standard in nuclear medicine for chronic osteomyelitis diagnosis is in vitro radiolabeled leukocytes. The long half-life of [111In] allows the localization of leukocytes over 48 hours. An investigation of multiple studies shows a decrease in sensitivity from 84% to 21% when

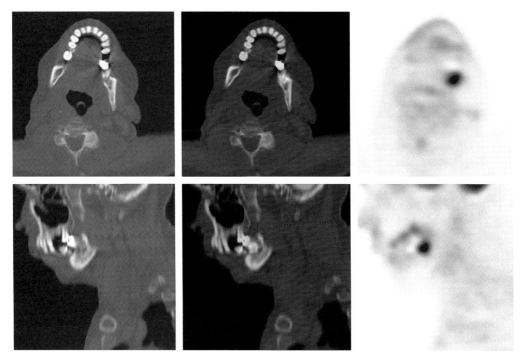

Fig. 7. PET CT of the mandible. Middle image is a fused PET CT for anatomical localization, a metabolically active lesion of increased FDG uptake. (*Courtesy of* Dr. Ronald Walker, Vanderbilt University, Nashville, TN.)

comparing the peripheral versus axial skeleton, however, which renders it unusable as a single modality for the maxillofacial region [34].

In a recent comparison of three-phase bone scintigraphy (single photon emission CT) and fluorodeoxyglucose-positron emission tomography in assessment of osteomyelitis of the jaws, the authors found a relatively low initial diagnostic sensitivity for positron emission tomography (64% versus 84%) [40]. The low specificity of single photon emission CT in surveillance led the authors to suggest that positron emission tomography follow-up screenings be performed as early as 1 month after surgery.

Treatment

Local delivery systems: nonresorbable

A gentamycin-polymethylmethacrylate (PMMA) delivery system for treatment of mandibular osteomyelitis was first introduced in 1978 (see Fig. 5) [41]. The release of aminoglycosides from these beads is of great conceptual benefit because local drug levels can be elevated while systemic nephrotoxic thresholds are not violated. When considering the cost and complications of long-term antibiotic treatment, it is not difficult to see the benefit of a local delivery that can greatly decrease treatment times. It has been found that the leaching characteristics of aminoglycosides from PMMA are the same in vascular and avascular tissues [42]. In animal orthopedic models, local delivery systems (gentamycin-PMMA) have shown a greater capacity to decrease CFU when compared with single-agent parenteral antibiotics administration [43]. Despite the benefits of local delivery systems, several shortcomings of PMMA have led investigators to look for other options. The elution from PMMA is unpredictable and never quite complete, they require a second surgery for removal, there are few heat-stable compatible antibiotic choices, and low-grade foreign body reactions are common [44] (Fig. 8). PMMA carriers are dense and compact, with one study showing 5.78% elution after 15 days and only 20% elution over the complete treatment course, which can lead to inadequate local release and subinhibitory antibiotic levels, sometimes with disturbing implications [45].

One study of PMMA-gentamycin bead placement characterized the recovery of "small colony variants" of *S aureus*, which are often antibiotic refractory [46]. With PMMA, antibiotics must

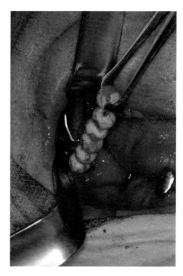

Fig. 8. Second surgery for removal of PMMA beads.

be water soluble, in powder form, and resistant to heat because of polymerization temperatures that can exceed 100°C. Recently, an alternative PMMA capsule containing tazocin (a water-insoluble, heat-labile aminoglycoside) was developed and tested in a rabbit osteomyelitis model [44]. After an 8-week treatment course, these capsules led to physical, radiographic, and histologic healing in these animals. The antibiotic selections have been extended by the authors to include amikacin, augmentin, cefotaxim, and clindamycin.

Local delivery systems: resorbable

Many biodegradable materials have been evaluated, including degradable polymers (polylactic acid, polyglycolic acid, polyparadioxanone), polyesters, hydroxyapatite and bioceramics, polymer-ceramic composites, calcium phosphates, fibrin sealant implants, and collagen sponges. Other than periodontal and hormonal applications, resorbable antibiotic systems have not been tested in humans [47]. The orthopedic and biomaterials research centers on induction of osteomyelitis in rabbit or rat tibias and in vitro carrier testing. Bioabsorbable systems have many advantages over nonresorbables. They do not require a second surgery for removal and, more importantly, they have a predictable local release of antibiotics. This elution follows first-order kinetics, in which the rate of release is proportional to the concentration of unreacted substance [47]. Theoretically, the rate of carrier degradation and antibiotic release can be tailored to coincide with anticipated osteomyelitis treatment times.

One well-designed study compared gentamycin-PMMA, gentamycin-collagen sponge, and parenteral cefazolin in a rat osteomyelitis model [43]. The local treatments outperformed the single-agent parenteral administration in reduction of S aureus CFUs. When comparing the two delivery systems, the gentamycin-collagen sponge reduced bacterial colony count to 1.4×10^2 CFU/g compared with 9.8×10^2 for the PMMA group. After 4 weeks of treatment with cefazolin and gentamycin-collagen sponge, 82% of sacrificed animals had no detectable bacteria in bone.

Many orthopedic studies involve easily prepared degradable cements that can fill bone defects. Hydroxyapatite cements (HAC) have a greater porosity than PMMA and can elute antibiotics at levels far above minimum bactericidal concentration over long periods of time. HAC is self-setting, isothermal, neutral pH, biocompatible, and bioabsorbable and commonly used for procedures such as cranioplasty. By replacing water with an appropriate antibiotic at the time of preparation, a convenient, moldable carrier can be fashioned. A recent in vitro and in vivo evaluation of an HAC-gentamycin delivery system showed promising results [48]. In treatment of rabbit tibial osteomyelitis, 6 weeks of HAC-gentamycin led to no culture growth of bone specimens taken from sacrificed animals. White blood cell counts precipitously declined and treatment group bony weights increased.

A similarly designed experiment assessed HAC usage with vancomycin [49]. The induced bone infections included methicillin-resistant S aureus and S aureus small colony variants verified at 3 weeks. The HAC-vancomycin group bone specimen, taken at day 42, showed no growth in culture and no histologic evidence of infection. The study was limited because of extremely high dosing of vancomycin (average 106.3 mg/kg), although serum levels stayed below toxic concentrations. An injectable calcium phosphate has been mixed with moxifloxacin and studied in regards to in vitro elution properties [50]. In comparison with acrylic, the release of moxifloxacin from the resorbable carrier was similar for the first 15 days yet stayed appreciably higher to an extreme of 450 days. Moxifloxacin, a new 6-fluoroquinolone, has good potential for treatment of chronic osteomyelitis because of broad-spectrum activity against gram-positive and -negative organisms, anaerobes, and even imipenem-resistant

bacterium such as B fragilis [51]. It has been shown to have excellent relative penetration into cortical and cancellous bone [52]. Calcium phosphate cements and fillers play a larger role in orthopedics for filling osseous defects. Because of the osteoconductive properties of calcium phosphate-antibiotic mixes, an average osseous filling of 91% was reported in a small study of six patients with long bone fractures [53].

Polymers such as polyglycolic acid and polylactic acid were first developed in the 1960s for use in maxillofacial surgery. Primarily because of poor mechanical properties, copolymers were developed, with the important advent of the polyglycolic acid–polylactic acid copolymer in a 90:10 ratio. The use of such polymers for drug delivery has been studied vigorously, but only in in vitro and in vivo animal models. The one consistent result in all studies was a high level of release from the carrier, regardless of the type of antibiotic used. Cefazolin and gentamycin were combined with polylactic acid/polyglycolic acid beads, releasing concentration above MIC for 2 to 4 weeks [54]. Similarly, ofloxacin was combined with polylactic-coglycolic acid, and 96% of the drug was released within 35 days [55]. A recent attempt to characterize the mass transport mechanism of drug release from polylactic-coglycolic acid found 91% dose elution over 30 days. They concluded that a 50:50 polylactic-coglycolic acid microparticle was ideal for efficient, sustained gentamycin release [56].

The promise of these studies of drug elution lies in the fact that treatment times may be reduced by high concentration local delivery, a clear advance over PMMA carriers. An in vivo investigation of polylactic acid delivery of ciprofloxacin in rabbit osteomyelitis yielded interesting results. The peak release of antibiotic occurred at day 190, whereas in vitro elution peaks were at day 100 [57]. Results suggested that a local therapy should be coupled to systemic antibiotic administration for the first 6 to 8 weeks of therapy for optimal results. It is currently unclear whether fluoroquinolones have a negative effect on bone healing, although it seems that relatively low concentrations (2.4 μg/mL) contributes to diminished healing of early stage fracture repair [58].

A new direction of the investigation into resorbable carriers is the use of polyesters of microbial origin. Polyhydroxybutyrate-based polyesters can be created through fermentation of certain bacteria. A recent study using a rabbit

osteomyelitis model looked at delivery of sulbac-
tam-ampicillin and sulbactam-cefoperazone from
polyhydroxybutyrate rods [59]. The emphasis was
on reducing any inflammatory response directed toward the degrading implant, which can be difficult
to characterize in an osteomyelitis environment.

Hyperbaric oxygen

The proposed mechanisms of action of hyperbaric oxygen (HBO) in the treatment of chronic
osteomyelitis are (1) reversal of wound hypoxia,
(2) enhancement of leukocyte killing, and (3)
direct killing of anaerobes and facultative anaerobes through the formation of oxygen radicals [7].
HBO also has been reported to augment the bactericidal effect of tobramycin against P aeruginosa
[60]. A systematic review of all literature assessing
HBO usage and wound healing stressed the overall lack of quality studies, most without control
groups [61]. Adverse events, such as vision
changes, seizures, pneumothorax, barotraumatic
otitis, and death, were reported in nine of the
included studies. Only two studies relating to
chronic osteomyelitis met the quality control
inclusion criteria for this 2003 review. Esterhai
and colleagues [62] studied use of HBO (two
ATM, 2-hour duration) on 28 patients with
chronic refractory osteomyelitis. This non-
randomized, controlled trial concluded that
HBO had no effect on length of hospitalization,
rate of wound repair, or recurrence of infection.
In a case series by David and colleagues [63], 34
of 38 patients remained free of recurrent osteomyelitis for an average of 34 months.

An attempt has been made to validate the use
of HBO for treatment of chronic osteomyelitis by
using a rabbit model [64]. No statistically significant differences were found in treatment groups
consisting of (1) antibiotic only, (2) HBO only,
and (3) antibiotic and HBO. The authors made
several interesting conclusions, asserting that
HBO is at least as effective as antibiotics in the
treatment of chronic osteomyelitis and that the
mechanism did not seem to be related to direct
antibacterial activity. Case-controlled studies
relating specifically to chronic osteomyelitis of
the jaws are virtually nonexistent. One case series
that investigated the treatment of 16 patients with
chronic osteomyelitis of the jaws showed a cure
rate of 44% [65]. The authors advocated antibiotics and surgery first and then considered HBO
in refractory patients and for patients with
chronic diffuse sclerosing osteomyelitis.

Recent antibiotic developments

The standard antibiotic regimen for chronic
osteomyelitis has been a 6-week course of the
appropriate agent given parenterally. Because of
high costs, inconvenience, and complications
associated with tunneled catheters, alternative
therapies have been devised and studied. Effective,
broad-coverage, highly absorbed oral antibiotics
would be ideal. Another common consideration is
the preponderance of antibiotic-resistant strains,
which were discussed earlier in this article. New
agents and multidrug protocols have been
developed to address these concerns.

Linezolid

Oxazolidinones are new synthetic antibiotics,
of which linezolid is a member. They are approved
for nosocomial pneumonia and complicated skin
infections. The mechanism of action is via inhibition of the 50s ribosomal subunit, thereby
impeding protein synthesis. Linezolid is significant
for strong action against gram-positive pathogens,
a 100% bioavailability after oral administration,
and good penetration into bone. There is a documented bacteriostatic effect against methicillin-
resistant S aureus, penicillin-resistant Streptococcus
sp, and vancomycin-resistant Enterococcus sp [9].

In a retrospective, noncontrolled study of 54
patients with orthopedic infections (not limited to
osteomyelitis) treated with linezolid, there was
a 90% clinical success rate [66]. Most patients
were given a 2-week course of parenteral vancomycin first, then linezolid was used for a variable
period that averaged 39 days. Although the results
of this study were positive, there was an 18% rate
of complications resulting in cessation of treatment. The most common causes were myelosup-
pression/anemia and intolerable gastrointestinal
upset. Another retrospective review of linezolid
efficacy consisted of 66 patients, all of whom suffered from chronic osteomyelitis [36]. Linezolid
was used alone or in combination for a cure rate
of 84.8%. Again, adverse effects led to discontinuation of treatment in 34.8% of patients, most of
whom had anemia. It must be remembered that
most of these patients were being treated for infections of a knee or hip prosthesis, leading to an
average treatment time of 14 weeks.

Linezolid has the potential to reduce hospital
admission stays by offering an oral "switch"
therapy. It should be reserved for the treatment
of drug-resistant pathogens or when glycopeptide
administration is not possible because of adverse

effects, resistance, allergy, or lack of intravenous access. Costs may be prohibitive, with the average wholesale cost for a 2-week course registering $1172 [67]. The reports of increasing resistance to vancomycin may tip interest toward the use of this oral antibiotic for the treatment of chronic osteomyelitis.

Tigecycline

Tigecycline is the first drug commercially available from a new class of antimicrobial agents, the glycylcyclines. This derivative of tetracycline is a parenteral, bacteriostatic drug with potential use in the fight against antibiotic-resistant organisms. This drug is active against multidrug-resistant, gram-positive and -negative organisms and anaerobes [68]. A comparison of tigecycline and vancomycin (± rifampin) in a rabbit osteomyelitis model was encouraging in respect to efficacy and bone penetration [69]. Tigecycline and rifampin were 100% successful in clearing bone samples of methicillin-resistant *S aureus*, whereas tigecycline and vancomycin alone were 90% effective. Because of structural modifications of tigecycline, it is not affected by the common forms of tetracycline resistance mechanisms (efflux pumps and ribosomal protection) [68]. The most common adverse events associated with tigecycline are nausea (43.2%), vomiting (26.7%), and diarrhea (12.7%), which leads to a 6.2% discontinuation rate [70].

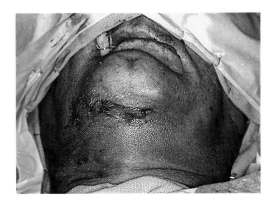

Fig. 10. Soft tissue damage from chronic fistulae.

Summary

The modern health care environment stresses short inpatient stays predicated on efficient, evidence-based protocols. Although there are relatively standard treatment approaches for chronic osteomyelitis, many avenues of investigation are being pursued to reflect contemporary concerns. The mainstays of care continue to include timely and thorough surgical débridement and culture-directed antibiotics, and resection/reconstruction when necessary (Figs. 9–11). Sensitive diagnostic screening is essential, and advances in radiology can lead to early confirmation of disease and accurate surveillance. There is potential to greatly reduce overall morbidity, chance of recurrent infection, and treatment courses by using the local delivery systems currently researched

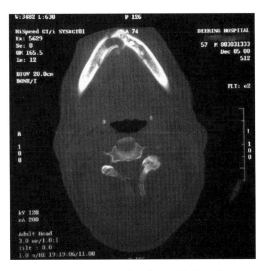

Fig. 9. CT examination of patient with chronic osteomyelitis secondary to dental implants. Cortical and medullary damage is clearly defined.

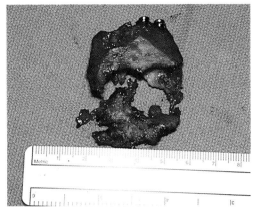

Fig. 11. Resection of anterior mandible shows sequestrum and devitalized bone adjacent to dental implants.

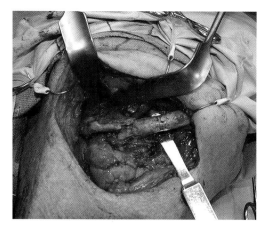

Fig. 12. When chronic infection is not controlled, frank fracture of the mandible is an eventuality.

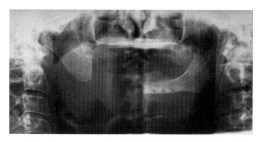

Fig. 13. A case of osteomyelitis that despite seemingly adequate resection margins has recurred. Sometimes the only recourse is removal of hardware and tracheostomy.

by orthopedic surgeons. The challenges posed by multidrug-resistant bacterium may be countered by sound culturing techniques and new antibiotics, never underestimating the potential morbidity associated with refractory bone infections (Figs. 12 and 13).

References

[1] Cierny G, Mader JT, Pennick JJ. A clinical staging system for adult osteomyelitis. Contemp Orthop 1985;10:17–37.
[2] Lew DP, Waldvogel FA. Osteomyelitis. N Engl J Med 1997;336:999–1007.
[3] Craigen MA, Watters J, Hackett JS. The changing epidemiology of osteomyelitis in children. J Bone Joint Surg Br 1992;74:541–5.
[4] Waldvogel FA, Medhoff G, Swartz MN. Osteomyelitis: a review of the clinical features, therapeutic consideration, and unusual aspect. N Engl J Med 1970;282:260–6.
[5] Asensi V, Valle E, Meana A, et al. In vivo interleukin-6 protects neutrophils from apoptosis in osteomyelitis. Infect Immun 2004;72(7):3823–8.
[6] Garcia-Alvarez F, Monzon M, Grasa JM, et al. Interleukin-1, interleukin-6, and interleukin-10 responses after antibiotic treatment in experimental chronic Staphylococcus aureus osteomyelitis. J Orthop Sci 2006;11:370–4.
[7] Marx RE. Chronic osteomyelitis of the jaws. Oral and Maxillofacial Clinics of North America 1991; 3(2):367–81.
[8] Calhoun KH, Shapiro RD, Stiernberg CM. Osteomyelitis of the mandible. Arch Head Neck Surg 1988;114:1157.
[9] Mader JT, Shirtliff ME, Bergquist SC, et al. Antimicrobial treatment of chronic osteomyelitis. Clin Orthop Relat Res 1999;360:47–65.
[10] Mercuri LG. Acute osteomyelitis of the jaws. Oral and Maxillofacial Clinics of North America 1991; 3(2):355–65.
[11] Marx RE, Carlson ER, Smith BR, et al. Isolation of Actinomyces species and Eikenella corrodens from patients with chronic diffuse sclerosing osteomyelitis. J Oral Maxillofac Surg 1994;52:26–33.
[12] Zuluaga AF, Galvis W, Saldarriaga JG, et al. Etiologic diagnosis of chronic osteomyelitis: a prospective study. Arch Intern Med 2006;166(1):95–100.
[13] Storoe W, Haug RH, Lillich TT. The changing face of odontogenic infections. J Oral Maxillofac Surg 2001;59:739–48.
[14] Koorbusch GF, Fotos P, Goll KT. Retrospective assessment of osteomyelitis. Oral Surg Oral Med Oral Pathol 1992;74:149–54.
[15] Scolozzi P, Lombardi T, Edney T, et al. Enteric bacteria mandibular osteomyelitis. Oral Surg Oral Med Oral Pathol Oral Radiol Endod 2005;99: E42–6.
[16] Robinson JL, Vaudry WL, Dobrovolsky W. Actinomycosis presenting as osteomyelitis in the pediatric population. Pediatr Infect Dis J 2005;24:365–9.
[17] Imamura M, Kakihara T, Yamamoto K, et al. Primary tuberculosis osteomyelitis of the mandible. Pediatr Int 2004;46:736–9.
[18] Bonomo RA, Szabo D. Mechanisms of multidrug resistance in Acinetobacter species and Pseudomonas aeruginosa. Clin Infect Dis 2006;43:S49–56.
[19] Howden BP, Ward PB, Charles P, et al. Treatment outcomes for serious infections caused by methicillin-resistant Staphylococcus aureus with reduced vancomycin susceptibility. Clin Infect Dis 2004;38: 521–8.
[20] Livermore DM. Interplay of impermeability and chromosomal B-lactamase activity in imipenem-resistant Pseudomonas aeruginosa. Antimicrob Agents Chemother 1992;36:2046–8.
[21] Deplano A, Denis O, Poirel L. Molecular characterization of an epidemic clone of panantibiotic-resistant Pseudomonas aeruginosa. J Clin Microbiol 2005;43:1198–204.

[22] Topazian RG, Goldberg MH, Hupp JR. Oral and maxillofacial infections. 4th edition. 2002. p. 215, 218.

[23] Wannfors K, Gazalius B. Blood flow in jaw bones affected by chronic osteomyelitis. Br J Oral Maxillofac Surg 1991;29(3):147–53.

[24] Dirschl DR, Almekinders LC. Osteomyelitis. Drugs 1993;45:29–43.

[25] Piattelli A, Cosci F, Scarano A, et al. Localized chronic suppurative bone infection as a sequel of peri-implantitis in a hydroxyapatite-coated dental implant. Biomaterials 1995;16:917–20.

[26] Votey SR. Diabetes mellitus, type 2: a review. Emedicine 2005.

[27] Aken'Ova YA, Bakare RA, Okunade MA, et al. Bacterial causes of acute osteomyelitis in sickle cell anaemia: changing infection profile. West Afr J Med 1995;14(4):255–8.

[28] Reinert S, Widlitzek H, Venderink DJ. The value of magnetic resonance imaging in the diagnosis of mandibular osteomyelitis. Br J Oral Maxillofac Surg 1999;37:459–63.

[29] Rohlin M. Diagnostic value of bone scintigraphy in osteomyelitis of the mandible. Oral Surg Oral Med Oral Path 1993;75:650–7.

[30] Flivik G, Sloth M, Rydholm U, et al. Technetium-99m nanocolloid scintigraphy in orthopedic infections: a comparison with In-111 labeled leukocytes. J Nucl Med 1993;34:1646–50.

[31] Tumeh SS, Aliabadi P, Weissman BN, et al. Disease activity in osteomyelitis: role of radiography. Radiology 1987;165:781–4.

[32] Kaim AH, Gross T, von Schulthess GK. Imaging of chronic posttraumatic osteomyelitis. Eur Radiol 2002;12:1193–202.

[33] Horger M, Eschmann SM, Pfannenberg C, et al. The value of SPET/CT in chronic osteomyelitis. Eur J Nucl Med Mol Imaging 2003;30(12):1665–73.

[34] Termaat MF, Raijmakers PGHM, Scholten HJ, et al. The accuracy of diagnostic imaging for the assessment of chronic osteomyelitis: a systematic review and meta-analysis. J Bone Joint Surg Am 2005;87:2464–71.

[35] Kaim A, Ledermann HP, Bongartz G, et al. Chronic posttraumatic osteomyelitis of the lower extremity: comparison of magnetic resonance imaging and combined bone scintigraphy/immunoscintigraphy with radiolabel led monoclonal antigranulocyte antibodies. Skeletal Radiol 2000;29:378–86.

[36] Senneville E, Legout L, Valette M, et al. Effectiveness and tolerability of prolonged linezolid treatment for chronic osteomyelitis: a retrospective study. Clin Ther 2006;28(8):1155–63.

[37] De Winter F, Van de Wiele C, Vogelaers D, et al. Flourine-18 fluorodeoxyglucose-positron emission tomography: a highly accurate imaging modality for the diagnosis of chronic musculoskeletal infections. J Bone Joint Surg Am 2001;83(5):651–60.

[38] Prandini N, Lazzeri E, Rossi B, et al. Nuclear medicine imaging of bone infections. Nucl Med Commun 2006;27:633–44.

[39] Zhuang HM, Loman JC, Cortes-Blanco A, et al. Hyperglycemia does not adversely affect FDG uptake by inflammatory and infectious lesions in FDG-PET imaging. J Nucl Med 2000;(Suppl 321).

[40] Hakim SG, Breuker CWR, Jacobsen HC, et al. The value of FDG-PET and bone scintigraphy with SPECT in the primary diagnosis and follow-up of patients with chronic osteomyelitis of the mandible. Int J Oral Maxillofac Surg 2006;35:809–16.

[41] Ludwig Von H, Haneke A. Ein neues verfahren in der behandlung der osteomyelitis. Dtsch Z Mund-Kiefer-Gesichts-Chir 1978;2:190–2.

[42] Alpert B, Colosi T, von Fraunhofer JA, et al. The in vivo behavior of gentamicin-PMMA beads in the maxillofacial region. J Oral Maxillofac Surg 1989; 47:46–9.

[43] Mendel V, Simanowski HJ, Scholz HC, et al. Therapy with gentamicin-PMMA beads, gentamicin-collagen sponge, and cefazolin for experimental osteomyelitis due to Staphylococcus aureus in rats. Arch Orthop Trauma Surg 2005;125:363–8.

[44] Borzsei L, Mintal T, Koos Z, et al. Examination of a novel, specified antibiotic therapy through polymethylmethacrylate capsules in a rabbit osteomyelitits model. Chemotherapy 2006;52:73–9.

[45] Bunetel L, Segui A, Cormier M, et al. Release of gentamycin from acrylic base cement. Clin Pharmacokinet 1989;17:271–97.

[46] von Eiff C, Bettin D, Proctor RA, et al. Recovery of small colony variants of Staphylococcus aureus following gentamycin bead placement for osteomyelitis. Clin Infect Dis 1997;25:1250–1.

[47] Garvin K, Feschuk C. Polylactide-polyglycolide antibiotic implants. Clin Orthop Relat Res 2005; 437:105–10.

[48] Joosten U, Joist A, Frebel T, et al. Evaluation of an in situ setting injectible calcium phosphate as a new carrier material for gentamicin in the treatment of chronic osteomyelitis: studies in vitro and in vivo. Biomaterials 2004;25:4287–95.

[49] Joosten U, Joist A, Gosheger G, et al. Effectiveness of hydroxyapatite-vancomycin bone cement in the treatment of Staphylococcus aureus induced chronic osteomyelitis. Biomaterials 2005;26:5251–8.

[50] Kanellakopoulou K, Tsaganos T, Athanassiou K, et al. Comparative elution of moxifloxacin from norian skeletal repair system and acrylic bone cement: an in vitro study. Biomaterials 2006;28: 217–20.

[51] Betriu C, Gomez M, Palau ML, et al. Activities of new antimicrobial agents against Bacteroides fragilis group: comparison with the activities of 14 other agents. Antimicrob Agents Chemother 1999;43(9): 2320–2.

[52] Malincarne L, Ghebregzabner M, Moretti MV, et al. Penetration of moxifloxacin into bone in patients

undergoing total knee arthroplasty. J Antimicrob Chemother 2006;57(5):950–4.

[53] Gitelis S, Brebach GT. The treatment of chronic osteomyelitis with a biodegradable antibiotic-impregnated implant. J Orthop Surg 2002;10:53–60.

[54] Wang G, Liu S, Ueng SW, et al. The release of cefazolin and gentamycin from biodegradable PLA/PGA beads. Int J Pharm 2004;273:203–12.

[55] Abazinge M, Jackson T, Yang Q, et al. Comparison of in vitro and in vivo release characteristics of sustained release ofloxacin microspheres. Drug Deliv 2000;7:77–81.

[56] Virto MR, Elorza B, Torrado S, et al. Improvement of gentamicin poly(D,L-lactic-co-glycolic acid) microspheres for treatment of osteomyelitis induced by orthopedic procedures. Biomaterials 2007;28:877–85.

[57] Koort JK, Suokas E, Veiranto M, et al. In vitro and in vivo testing of bioabsorbable antibiotic containing bone filler for osteomyelitis treatment. J Biomed Mater Res A 2006;10:532–40.

[58] Huddleston PM, Steckelberg JM, Hanssen AD, et al. Ciprofloxacin inhibition of experimental fracture healing. J Bone Joint Surg Am 2000;82:161–73.

[59] Korkusuz F, Korkusuz P, Eksioglu F, et al. In vivo response to biodegradable controlled antibiotic release systems. J Biomed Mater Res 2001;55(2):217–28.

[60] Mader JT, Adams KR, Wallace WR, et al. Hyperbaric oxygen as adjunctive therapy for osteomyelitis. Infect Dis Clin North Am 1990;4(3):433–40.

[61] Wang C, Schwaitzberg S, Berliner E, et al. Hyperbaric oxygen for treating wounds: a systematic review of the literature. Arch Surg 2003;138:272–9.

[62] Esterhai JL, Pisarello J, Brighton CT, et al. Adjunctive hyperbaric oxygen therapy in the treatment of chronic refractory osteomyelitis. J Trauma 1987; 27(7):763–8.

[63] Davis JC, Hechman JD, DeLee JC, et al. Chronic nonhematogenous osteomyelitis treated with adjunct hyperbaric oxygen. J Bone Joint Surg Am 1986;68:1210–7.

[64] Mader JT, Guckian JC, Glass DL, et al. Therapy with hyperbaric oxygen for the experimental osteomyelitis due to Staphylococcus aureus in rabbits. J Infect Dis 1978;138(3):312–8.

[65] Van Merkesteyn JP, Bakker DJ, Van der Waal I, et al. Hyperbaric oxygen treatment of chronic osteomyelitis of the jaws. Int J Oral Surg 1984;13(5): 386–95.

[66] Harwood PJ, Talbot C, Dimoutsos M, et al. Early experience with linezolid for infections in orthopedics. Injury Int J Care Injured 2006;37:818–26.

[67] Shuford JA, Steckelberg JM. Role of oral antimicrobial therapy in the management of osteomyelitis. Curr Opin Infect Dis 2003;16:515–9.

[68] Rose W, Rybak MJ. Tigecycline: first of a new class of antimicrobial agents. Pharmacotherapy 2006; 26(8):1099–110.

[69] Yin LY, Lazzarini L, Li F, et al. Comparative evaluation of tigecycline and vancomycin, with and without rifampicin, in the treatment of methicillin-resistant Staphylococcus aureus experimental osteomyelitis in a rabbit model. J Antimicrob Chemother 2005;55:995–1002.

[70] Saccidanand S, Penn RL, Embil JM. Efficacy and safety of tigecycline monotherapy compared with vancomycin plus aztreonam in patients with complicated skin and skin structure infections. Int J Infect Dis 2005;9:251–61.

ELSEVIER
SAUNDERS

Oral Maxillofacial Surg Clin N Am 19 (2007) 535–551

ORAL AND
MAXILLOFACIAL
SURGERY CLINICS
of North America

Bone Morphogenetic Proteins: A Realistic Alternative to Bone Grafting for Alveolar Reconstruction

Ulf M.E. Wikesjö, DDS, DMD, PhD*, Yi-Hao Huang, DDS, MS,
Giuseppe Polimeni, DDS, MS, Mohammed Qahash, DDS, MS

*Laboratory for Applied Periodontal & Craniofacial Regeneration, Medical College of Georgia
School of Dentistry AD1430, 1120 15th Street, Augusta, GA 30912, USA*

Common complications encountered when replacing missing teeth using endosseous oral implants include severely resorbed alveolar ridges after long-term edentulism or alveolar ridges compromised from advanced periodontal disease or trauma, which disallow implant placement to meet aesthetic and functional demands. Conversely, placing oral implants to optimally meet aesthetic and functional demands in sites that exhibit alveolar ridge aberrations often results in exposure of the implant bone-anchoring surface. Clinicians commonly attempt to overcome alveolar ridge aberrations by augmenting anticipated implant sites using bone biomaterials that originate from allogeneic or xenogeneic cadaver sources (bone derivatives) or using synthetic biomaterials (bone substitutes) (Box 1). Such bone biomaterials have been used as stand-alone therapies and in combinations, also including grafting using autologous bone. Nonresorbable and bioresorbable barrier membranes have been used to contain implanted biomaterials. Nonresorbable barriers, usually expanded polytetrafluoroethylene (ePTFE) membranes or titanium mesh, must be removed in a second surgical procedure. Barrier membranes also have been used without bone biomaterials in support of osteogenic (local) bone formation—a treatment concept known as guided bone regeneration (GBR). An increasing body of evidence suggests that bone biomaterials may delay or interfere with osteogenic bone formation because of slow resorption rates and may compromise the quality of bone for implant placement and retention. This may be reflected in decreased success or survival rates for oral implants placed in augmented sites compared with implants placed into nonaugmented sites. Patients have become increasingly concerned about the use of biomaterials derived from human or animal cadaver sources for elective procedures, including implant dentistry, because of potential risk of disease transmission.

Bone morphogenetic proteins

Polypeptide growth factors are biologic mediators that regulate cellular activities, including cell migration, proliferation, differentiation, and matrix synthesis. Over the last decades, there has been a focused effort to add to the knowledge of how polypeptide growth factors may influence repair or regeneration of tissues. These native ligands have been shown to have pleiotropic effects that support regeneration in several settings and accelerate healing processes. They exert their effects by binding to specific cell membrane receptors and initiate complex cascades eventually reaching a nuclear target gene to generate signals for specific phenotype expression. Examples of polypeptide growth factors in bone, cementum, and healing tissues include platelet-derived growth factor (PDGF), vascular endothelial growth factor (VGF),

Earlier versions of this text have been published for reviews in journals and book chapters. The text is continuously subject to revisions and updating as new information becomes available in our laboratory. The Laboratory for Applied Periodontal & Craniofacial Regeneration is supported in part by a grant from Nobel Biocare AB, Sweden.

* Corresponding author.

E-mail address: uwikesjo@mail.mcg.edu (U.M.E. Wikesjö).

1042-3699/07/$ - see front matter © 2007 Elsevier Inc. All rights reserved.
doi:10.1016/j.coms.2007.07.004

oralmaxsurgery.theclinics.com

Box 1. Bone grafts, bone biomaterials, and biologics

Grafts
  Autogenous bone; fresh/frozen
  Allogeneic bone; fresh/frozen (not used in dentistry)
  Xenogeneic bone; fresh/frozen (not used in dentistry)
  Osteoblast cell constructs (experimental)

Biomaterials
  Bone derivatives (processed cadaver bone)
    Allogeneic bone implants
      (decalcified) freeze-dried allogeneic bone (DFDBA/FDBA)
    Xenogeneic bone implants
      deproteinized bovine bone mineral (BioCera™, BBP®, Bio-Oss®)
      $CaCO_3$ coral exoskeleton (Biocoral®)
  Bone substitutes ("synthetic bone")
    Ceramics
      β-tricalcium phosphate (β-TCP)
      hydroxyapatite (HA)
      Ca_2SO_4 (plaster of Paris)
      calcium phosphate cements (Ceredex™, α-BSM®)
      bioactive glass (PerioGlas®, BioGran®)
    Polymers
      methylmethacrylate (HTR Synthetic Bone)
      poly-α-hydroxy acids (PLA, PLGA)

Biologics
  Growth factors (PDGF, TGF-β, IGF-1, VEGF)
  Differentiation factors (BMP-2, OP-1, GDF-5, GDF-7)
  Matrix factors (fibronectin, vitronectin, thrombospondin-1)
  Peptides (thrombin peptide TP508)
  Small molecules (PGE receptor antagonists)
  Platelet-Rich-Plasma

Combinations

---

transforming growth factor-α and -β (TGF-α, TGF-β), epidermal growth factor (EGF), insulin-like growth factors-I and -II (IGF-I, IGF-II), cementum derived growth factor (CGF), parathyroid hormone-related protein (PTHrP), bone morphogenetic proteins (BMPs), tumor necrosis factor (TNF), monocyte-derived growth factors (MDGF), and acidic and basic fibroblast factor (aFGF, bFGF)[1,2].

In 1965, Dr. Marshall Urist reported the discovery that bone matrix preparations induced cartilage, bone, and marrow formation when implanted subcutaneously and intramuscularly in rodent models [3,4]. The responsible proteins, BMPs, were identified [5–7] after extensive purification and molecular cloning [8–10]. Most BMPs comprise three portions: signal peptide, propeptide, and mature region. The propeptide and mature region contains seven conserved cysteine

residues characteristic of the TGF-β superfamily. Ever since, BMPs have been studied extensively and represent a significant addition to the understanding of bone biology and development. The influence of BMPs may begin as early as at gastrulation to continue throughout postfetal life recapitulating processes in embryonic bone formation [11]. BMPs act as growth and differentiation factors and as chemotactic agents. BMPs stimulate angiogenesis and migration, proliferation, and differentiation of mesenchymal stem cells into cartilage- and bone-forming cells in an area of bone injury. Currently, more than 20 BMPs have been identified, several of which induce bone formation.

Extracts from the collagenous matrix of bone include BMPs but also other growth factors. The yield of extracted and partially purified BMPs only amounts to 1 μg/kg fresh bone, which makes it difficult to obtain sufficient quantities to evaluate a therapeutic potential in clinically relevant skeletal defects [12]. Recombinant technologies have been used to produce BMPs. Because the structures of several human BMPs have been identified, it is possible to use DNA probes to obtain the human cDNA sequence. The human cDNA is cloned and spliced into a viral expression vector. Chinese hamster ovary cells and *Escherichia coli* transfected to become carriers have been used to produce BMPs in large quantities for preclinical and clinical evaluation [13,14]. Recombinant human BMP (rhBMP) produced in this fashion provides optimal compatibility for clinical application without potential immunologic reactions or transmission of infectious material inherent in technologies that rely on purified extracts from human or animal cadaver sources [15,16].

rhBMP-2, recombinant human osteogenic protein-1 (rhOP-1/rhBMP-7), and recombinant human growth/differentiation factor-5 (rhGDF-5) are currently being pursued as therapies for reconstruction and repair of induced and congenital skeletal defects and have been evaluated for indications such as spine fusion, hip arthroplasty, and fracture repair [17–27]. rhBMP-2, rhOP-1, and rhGDF-5 technologies also have been evaluated for craniofacial indications, including segmental resection defects, plastic procedures, and congenital defects [28–47]. Still other studies have explored the potential clinical use of BMPs for alveolar augmentation [48–59], sinus lift procedures [60–73], implant fixation [74–89], and periodontal regeneration [90–108]. rhBMP-2 and rhOP-1/rhBMP-7 have been approved for orthopedic indications and introduced to clinical practice, with rhBMP-2 most recently being approved for craniofacial indications (Box 2).

Bone morphogenetic protein delivery systems

Several matrices or delivery systems have been examined to evaluate their efficacy and biocompatibility as carriers for BMPs. For this text, of specific interest are biomaterials that have been evaluated for craniofacial indications using large animal models. These materials include particulate and putty formulations of inorganic biomaterials from natural or synthetic sources based on hydroxyapatite [48,74,100], β-tricalcium phosphate [66], calcium sulphates/plaster of Paris [109], calcium phosphates [56,87,102], calcium carbonates [74], and bioglass technologies [49] and organic

---

Box 2. BMPs approved for clinical use and indications

rhBMP-2 (*Wyeth/Medtronic*)
InductOs® (CHMP approved)
  Open tibia fracture, 2002
  Interbody spinal fusion, 2005
INFUSE® Bone Graft (FDA approved)
  Interbody spinal fusion, 2002
  Open tibia fracture, 2004
  Oral/maxillofacial, 2007

rhOP-1 (*Stryker*)
OP-1® Implant (FDA HDE & CHMP approved)
  Recalcitrant long bone nonunions, 2001/2004
OP-1® Putty (FDA HDE approved)
  Osterolateral (intertransverse) lumbar spinal fusion revision, 2004

---

polymers, including allogeneic/xenogeneic collagen preparations [49,52,75,92,97,100], hyaluronan [52,105], poly-α-hydroxy acids [74,93,94,98,100], and methylmethacrylate [74]. Biomaterials have been used alone or in combination, also including autogenous bone and fibrin clots [100]. BMP preparations have been used in conjunction with occlusive or porous, resorbable or nonresorbable, space-providing devices/membranes for GBR [53,81,88,89,106,107]. Requirements for structural properties of a carrier material depend on the particular indication, inlay or onlay, and whether to use an implantable or injectable minimally invasive approach. It is essential for any carrier material to maintain its physical integrity at the target site while releasing BMP to desired concentration over time. At the same time, it should resorb in a timely fashion so as not to obstruct bone formation or remain in situ to potentially compromise physiologic and biomechanical properties of bone.

An absorbable collagen sponge (ACS) was the first FDA-approved BMP carrier technology (see Box 2). ACS is a bovine type I collagen matrix that is soak-loaded with a BMP solution before surgical implantation. The rhBMP-2/ACS construct has shown clinical efficacy for several indications; however, it may become vulnerable to tissue compression and seems less effective for onlay indications. ACS has been combined with various biomaterials, including hydroxyapatite and bioglass technologies, organic polymers, including allogeneic/xenogeneic bone collagen matrices, or space-providing occlusive or porous, resorbable, or nonresorbable devices potentially providing structural integrity [48,49,53,75,76,81, 88,89,106,107]. ACS provides a bolus or near-bolus release of BMP upon implantation. Various other carrier technologies providing other release kinetics and structural properties have been evaluated in the search for technologies for onlay indications and technologies for injectable minimally invasive procedures. Putty consistency calcium phosphate cements that set to into noncompressible implants with apparently different release kinetics have shown considerable promise [87,102]. Calcium phosphate cements can be used as implantable and injectable technologies providing opportunity for minimal invasive procedures.

An intriguing concept of applying BMPs onto titanium surfaces for enhanced local bone formation and osseointegration has been evaluated in rodent and canine ectopic or orthotopic models [110–117]. Direct cellular approaches and molecular signaling also are being considered. BMPs produced by cells at the site of repair have been tested using cDNA vector systems, which include viral delivery (in vivo/ex vivo) and direct cDNA

delivery at the site [118]. Safety seems to be a concern with such cell-based technologies.

Applications in maxillofacial surgery and periodontics

Several studies have evaluated BMP technologies for alveolar augmentation and endosseous implant osseointegration. The following section focuses on critical advances that demonstrate the remarkable biologic and clinical potential that BMPs may bring to dentoalveolar rehabilitation, including osseointegration of oral implants.

rhBMP-2/ACS

Using a discriminating canine model [119], our laboratory first demonstrated that a BMP construct used as an onlay has the potential to induce clinically relevant alveolar bone augmentation and osseointegration [83]. Ten-millimeter endosseous implants were inserted 5 mm into the surgically reduced edentulous mandibular alveolar ridge to create critical-sized, 5-mm, supra-alveolar peri-implant defects. rhBMP-2/ACS or buffer/ACS (control) was draped over the exposed

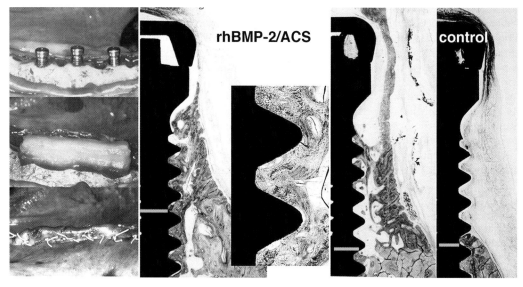

Fig. 1. Critical-sized, 5-mm, supra-alveolar peri-implant defect treated with rhBMP-2/ACS or ACS without rhBMP-2 (control). Clinical photographs show the supra-alveolar defect implanted with rhBMP-2/ACS before and after wound closure for primary intention healing. The left photomicrographs show defect sites having received rhBMP-2/ACS exhibiting bone formation reaching or exceeding the implant platform, the newly formed bone showing osseointegration to the machined titanium implant surface (*high magnification insert*). Control sites show limited, if any, bone formation. Green lines delineate the level of the surgically reduced alveolar crest. Healing interval, 16 weeks. (*Modified from* Sigurdsson TJ, Fu E, Tatakis DN, et al. Bone morphogenetic protein-2 enhances peri-implant bone regeneration and osseointegration. Clin Oral Implants Res 1997;8:367–74; with permission.)

implants in contralateral jaw quadrants and the defects sites were closed advancing and suturing the mucoperiosteal flaps for primary intention healing (Fig. 1). The implant sites were subjected to histometric evaluation after a 16-week healing interval. Sites that received rhBMP-2 revealed significant bone formation, including osseointegration along the exposed implant surface. Newly formed bone approached or exceeded the implant platform, whereas controls showed limited, if any, bone formation. However, there was significant variability in bone formation; rhBMP-2–induced bone made up only a thin layer covering the implant surface in several sites. Apparently the ACS carrier was ineffective in consistently producing a space for adequate rhBMP-2–induced bone formation.

These observations become even more conspicuous when compared with observations in the same preclinical model evaluating decalcified, freeze-dried, allogeneic bone (DFDBA) combined with GBR or GBR alone [120], both treatment concepts significant to modern clinical practice (Fig. 2). Again using a canine model, contralateral, critical-sized, 5-mm, supra-alveolar peri-implant defects, each including two endosseous implants, received a space-providing ePTFE membrane for GBR and DFDBA rehydrated in autologous blood or the ePTFE membrane alone. The implant sites were subjected to histometric evaluation after a 16-week healing interval. The type

I collagen DFDBA biomaterial remained apparently unaltered in all sites that received this treatment and exhibited no signs of biodegradation. The DFDBA particles appeared solidified within a dense connective tissue matrix and in close contact to the titanium implant surface without evidence of bone formation and osseointegration. Overall, bone formation along the implant surface was limited and clinically irrelevant for both treatments—GBR/DFDBA and GBR alone. Notably, physiologic concentrations of bone growth factors and BMPs sequestered in the DFDBA matrix apparently had no relevant effect on alveolar bone formation, because the DFDBA particles were invested in fibrous connective tissue without evidence of any bone metabolic activity. In contrast to results observed for the rhBMP-2 protocol, the results from this study suggested that DFDBA has no relevant osteoinductive, osteoconductive, or other adjunctive effect to GBR and that GBR technologies have limited potential to support osteogenesis (augment alveolar bone), at least for onlay indications.

rhBMP-2/ACS as a stand-alone therapy is associated with concerning weaknesses, in particular for onlay indications. Lack of structural integrity disallows predictable bone volumes, and the newly formed bone is sparsely trabecular, which likely bars placement of endosseous implants within 8 weeks after augmentation using staged protocols (Fig. 3) [83,86]. To overcome

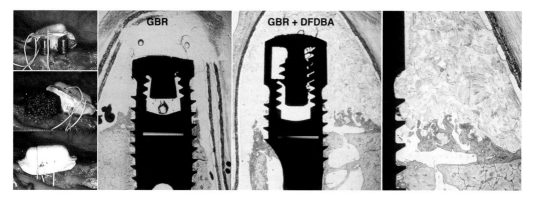

Fig. 2. Critical-sized, 5-mm, supra-alveolar peri-implant defect treated with GBR (occlusive space-providing ePTFE membrane; *green arrowheads*) with or without DFDBA. The clinical panels show the supra-alveolar defect with the GBR membrane, with DFDBA rehydrated in autologous blood, and with the membrane in place before wound closure for primary intention healing. Note limited regeneration of alveolar bone in absence and presence of DFDBA, which suggests that (1) the innate regenerative potential of alveolar bone is limited and (2) the DFDBA biomaterial has limited, if any, osteoinductive and/or osteoconductive properties to support bone regeneration. Green lines delineate the level of the surgically reduced alveolar crest. Healing interval, 16 weeks. (*From* Caplanis N, Sigurdsson TJ, Rohrer MD, et al. Effect of allogeneic, freeze-dried, demineralized bone matrix on guided bone regeneration in supra-alveolar peri-implant defects in dogs. Int J Oral Maxillofac Implants 1997;12:634–42; with permission.)

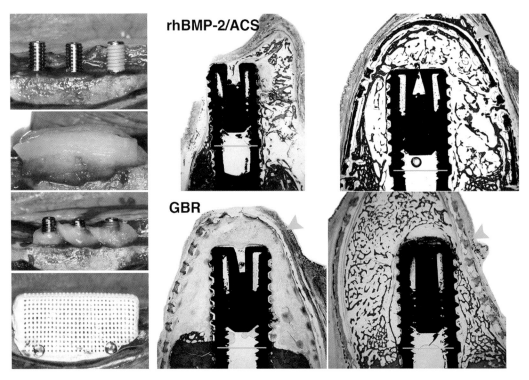

Fig. 3. Critical-sized, 5-mm, supra-alveolar peri-implant defects treated with rhBMP-2/ACS, GBR, or rhBMP-2/ACS combined with GBR using a porous, space-providing ePTFE membrane. The clinical panels show the supra-alveolar defect with rhBMP-2/ACS and with the porous GBR membrane. Note how rhBMP-2–induced bone fills the space provided by the membrane (*green arrowheads*), whereas rhBMP-2/ACS alone provides irregular bone formation (*top left*). GBR alone (*bottom left*) provides for limited, if any, regeneration of alveolar bone. Green lines delineate the level of the surgically reduced alveolar crest. Healing interval, 8 weeks. (*Modified from* Wikesjö UME, Qahash M, Thomson RC, et al. Space-providing expanded polytetrafluoroethylene devices define alveolar augmentation at dental implants induced by recombinant human bone morphogenetic protein-2. Clin Implant Dent Relat Res 2003;5:112–23; Wikesjö UME, Qahash M, Thomson RC, et al. rhBMP-2 significantly enhances guided bone regeneration. Clin Oral Implants Res 2004;15:194–204; with permission.)

structural limitations, rhBMP-2/ACS has been sandwiched with various bone biomaterials to enhance its structural integrity in support of bone formation [1,2]. Although supporting larger bone volumes, the long-term integrity of such induced bone formation is questioned because of compromises commonly associated with the bone biomaterials including, but not limited to, slow or no bioresorption that compromises biomechanical properties of bone or inflammatory reactions associated with bone biomaterials degradation resulting in local bone resorption [48,49,100].

Subsequent studies evaluated a space-providing, porous ePTFE device to support rhBMP-2/ACS–induced bone formation. The concept behind the design was to provide an unobstructed space to obviate compression of the rhBMP-2/ACS construct and simultaneously allow vascular and cellular elements from the gingival connective tissue

to support rhBMP-2–induced bone formation (Fig. 3). Bilateral, critical-sized, 5-mm, supra-alveolar peri-implant defects were created in a canine model [88,89]. Four animals received the space-providing, dome-shaped, porous ePTFE device alone or combined with rhBMP-2/ACS in contralateral jaw quadrants, and four animals received rhBMP-2/ACS solo versus rhBMP-2/ACS combined with the porous ePTFE device in contralateral jaw quadrants. The implant sites were subjected to histometric analysis after an 8-week healing interval. Similar to that observed in our previous studies [83,86,119], GBR limitedly enhanced bone formation [89]. Jaw quadrants that received rhBMP-2/ACS alone showed significant augmentation of the alveolar ridge; however, the height and volume of the induced bone were highly irregular [88]. In contrast, the dome-shaped, space-providing, porous ePTFE device–rhBMP-2/ACS combination predictably resulted in bone formation filling the large space provided by the device [88,89]. The newly formed bone interacted with the oral implants to generate osseointegration. This study provided important insight into tissue engineering principles using BMPs. BMP bone formation follows the outline of a space or matrix; in other words, you may outline the geometry of the newly formed bone already in the design of the matrix.

In still other studies, rhBMP-2 constructs have been evaluated for inlay indications using intrabony defect models. Jovanovic and colleagues [53] showed rhBMP-2/ACS to be an effective treatment when implanted into space-providing alveolar ridge defects. Combining rhBMP-2/ACS with GBR provided no additional value. Surgically created, mandibular, alveolar ridge, full-thickness, 15- × 10-mm, saddle-type defects in a canine model were randomly assigned to receive rhBMP-2/ACS, rhBMP-2/ACS combined with GBR, or control treatments. The GBR protocol used traditional occlusive ePTFE devices. Histometric evaluation followed a 12-week healing interval. Postsurgery complications included wound failure in as many as 44% of the sites receiving the occlusive ePTFE device with or without rhBMP-2. The histometric analysis revealed bone fill averaging 101% for defects that received rhBMP-2/ACS or rhBMP-2/ACS combined with GBR (without wound failure) and 92% for defects that received GBR alone

(without wound failure). Bone fill for the surgical control averaged 60%.

The observations above demonstrate that rhBMP-2 may be used to augment alveolar bone when used as an onlay and as an inlay. The observations also point to the importance of space provision for rhBMP-2–induced bone formation. Supra-alveolar defects (onlay indications), such as the critical-sized peri-implant defect model, may require rhBMP-2 constructs exhibiting structural integrity providing space for alveolar augmentation or should be combined with suitable space-providing devices for optimal bone formation. In contrast, space-providing intrabony defects (inlay indications) such as the saddle-type defect may be treated successfully using rhBMP-2 constructs of lesser structural integrity. The addition of occlusive GBR devices does not provide additional value to the rhBMP-2 technology. Notably, occlusive GBR devices may readily become exposed, thereby overall compromising wound healing.

Alternative delivery technologies

Two recent studies have evaluated BMP technologies that exhibit structural integrity for onlay indications. A first study showed that rhBMP-2 in a DFDBA/fibrin carrier might have substantial clinical use to augment demanding alveolar ridge defects allowing placement and osseointegration of oral implants [84]. Using a canine model, bilateral,

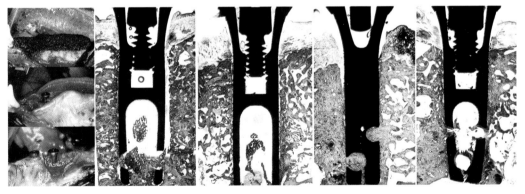

Fig. 4. Surgically created horizontal alveolar ridge defect implanted with rhBMP-2 combined with DFDBA rehydrated in autologous blood. The clinical panels show the rhBMP-2/DFDBA/fibrin construct placed onto the surgically reduced flat alveolar ridge before wound closure for primary intention healing. Transmucosal oral titanium implants were placed into the rhBMP-2–induced alveolar ridge at weeks 8 and 16 after surgery. The animals were euthanized 24 weeks after the ridge augmentation procedure. The left photomicrographs show implants placed at week 8 and the right photomicrographs show implants placed at week 16. Approximately 90% of the bone-anchoring surface of the implants was housed in rhBMP-2–induced bone, which exhibited limited evidence of crestal resorption. There was no significant difference in bone density between rhBMP-2–induced and contiguous resident bone. Also osseointegration (approximately 55%) was similar in induced and resident bone regardless of whether the implants were placed at week 8 or 16. (*Modified from* Sigurdsson TJ, Nguyen S, Wikesjö UME. Alveolar ridge augmentation with rhBMP-2 and bone to implant contact in induced bone. Int J Periodontics Restorative Dent 2001;21:461–73; with permission.)

critical-sized, horizontal alveolar ridge defects received an rhBMP-2/DFDBA/fibrin onlay. Non-submerged, 10-mm titanium implants were placed into the rhBMP-2–induced alveolar ridge at 8 and 16 weeks (Fig. 4). The implant sites were subject to a histometric evaluation at 24 weeks post surgery. Approximately 90% of the bone-anchoring surface of the implants was invested in rhBMP-2–induced bone. Similar levels of bone implant contact (approximately 55%) were observed in induced and resident bone regardless of osseointegration interval (8 or 16 weeks). There was no significant difference in bone density between rhBMP-2–induced and resident bone, which emphasized the clinical potential of this rhBMP-2 composite. However, the use of cadaver-sourced biomaterials, including DFDBA, may have difficulty being publicly accepted, thus synthetic carrier technologies for alveolar indications need to be explored.

The second study evaluated a synthetic carrier technology and showed that implantation of rhBMP-2 in a calcium phosphate cement matrix (α-BSM) seems to be an effective protocol for alveolar ridge augmentation and immediate osseointegration (Fig. 5) [87]. Again using a canine model, critical-sized, 5-mm, supraalveolar, peri-implant defects were used. Three animals received rhBMP-2/α-BSM in contralateral jaw quadrants (rhBMP-2 at 0.40 and 0.75 mg/mL). Three additional animals received α-BSM alone (control). The defect sites were subjected to histometric evaluation after a 16-week healing interval. rhBMP-2/

α-BSM induced clinically relevant augmentation of the alveolar ridge. Control sites exhibited limited, if any, bone formation. Vertical bone augmentation comprised almost the entire 5-mm exposed implant, the newly formed bone exhibiting bone density approximating 60% (type II bone) with established cortex and bone-implant contact approximating 27%. This novel technology shows considerable promise for several clinical indications because α-BSM may be shaped to desirable contour and sets to provide space for rhBMP-2–induced bone formation. α-BSM is injectable for inlay and minimally invasive indications and may prove to be a formidable technology for augmentation of the maxillary sinus in conjunction with placement of oral implants in the posterior maxilla, predictably pin-pointing bone formation at the implant body.

Peri-implantitis and reosseointegration

Research also has shown that rhBMP-2 supports significant reosseointegration of endosseous implants exposed to peri-implantitis [79]. Ligature-induced peri-implantitis lesions were created around hydroxyapatite-coated titanium implants in the posterior mandible and maxilla over 11 months in a nonhuman primate model. Induced peri-implantitis lesions exhibited a microbiota similar to that of advanced human peri-implantitis and periodontal disease and complex defect morphology. At reconstruction, the

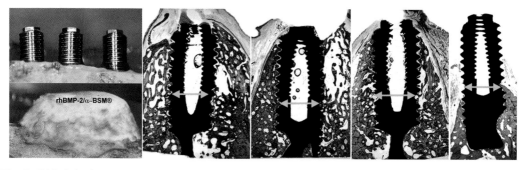

Fig. 5. Critical-sized, 5-mm, supra-alveolar peri-implant defect treated with rhBMP-2 in a calcium phosphate cement (α-BSM) or α-BSM without rhBMP-2 (control). The clinical panels show the supra-alveolar peri-implant defect before and after application of α-BSM. The photomicrographs show representative observations for jaw quadrants receiving rhBMP-2/α-BSM, in this particular jaw quadrant rhBMP-2 at 0.4 mg/mL. Note substantial new bone formation at sites treated with rhBMP-2/α-BSM compared with the control (*far right*) exhibiting limited, if any, evidence of new bone formation. The rhBMP-2–induced bone exhibits similar trabeculation, osseointegration, and cortex formation as the contiguous resident bone. Also note no evidence of residual biomaterial. Green arrows delineate the apical extension of the supra-alveolar peri-implant defects. Healing interval, 16 weeks. (*Modified from* Wikesjö UME, Sorensen RG, Kinoshita A, et al. rhBMP-2/α-BSM induces significant vertical alveolar ridge augmentation and dental implant osseointegration. Clin Implant Dent Relat Res 2002;4:173–81; with permission.)

defect sites were surgically debrided and the implant surfaces cleaned before surgical placement of rhBMP-2/ACS. Control defects received buffer/ACS. Histometric analysis performed after a 16-week healing interval revealed clinically relevant threefold greater vertical bone gain in sites that received rhBMP-2 compared with control. Importantly, rhBMP-2–treated sites exhibited convincing evidence of reosseointegration (Fig. 6). The results from this challenging nonhuman primate model suggest that surgical implantation of rhBMP-2 may have considerable clinical use in the reconstruction of peri-implantitis defects and alveolar defects of lesser complexity.

Functional loading of rhBMP-2–induced bone

A critical test for any technology aimed at alveolar augmentation in support of osseointegration of endosseous implants is functional loading. A recent study established that rhBMP-2 induces normal physiologic bone, which allows installation, osseointegration, and long-term functional loading of endosseous implants [81]. Mandibular, alveolar ridge, full-thickness, 15- × 10-mm, saddle-type defects were surgically created in a canine model. The defect sites were immediately implanted with rhBMP-2/ACS. Healing was allowed to progress for 12 weeks when endosseous oral implants were placed into rhBMP-2–induced and adjoining resident bone (control) (Fig. 7). After 16 weeks of osseointegration, the implants received abutments and prosthetic reconstruction. The reconstructed implants were exposed to

functional loading for 12 months when the implant sites were subjected to histometric analysis. The rhBMP-2–induced bone exhibited features of the resident bone, including a re-established cortex. Implants exposed to functional loading for 12 months exhibited some crestal resorption. The implants exhibited a mean bone contact that approximated respectable 50% in rhBMP-2–induced and 75% in resident bone. There were no significant differences between implants placed into rhBMP-2–induced and resident bone for any parameter evaluated. The implant sites exhibited some crestal resorption and clinically relevant osseointegration, which supported functional loading over 12 months. Although previously reported studies convincingly demonstrated clinically relevant alveolar bone augmentation and implant osseointegration after surgical implantation of rhBMP-2, this study first showed the functional use of rhBMP-2–induced bone in implant dentistry.

Clinical studies evaluating bone morphogenetic proteins

Case reports, case series, and randomized controlled trials evaluating BMP technologies for craniofacial clinical indications have focus on sinus and alveolar ridge augmentation, and reconstruction of congenital or induced discontinuity defects [33,34,45,51,54,60,62,63,74,77,78].

Sinus augmentation

Three reports concern application of rhOP-1 in a demineralized bovine bone matrix carrier

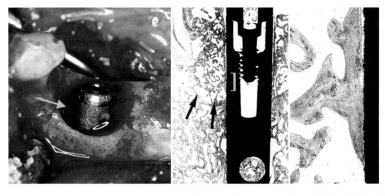

Fig. 6. Re-osseointegration after treatment of chronic peri-implantitis defect with rhBMP-2/ACS. The clinical panel shows the debrided peri-implantitis defect before treatment with rhBMP-2/ACS; the green arrow points to the aspect of the implant shown in the photomicrographs. Black arrows delineate the apical aspect of the peri-implantitis defect; the green bracket depicts a high magnification area (*right*) showing re-osseointegration. Note that the rhBMP-2–induced bone exhibits qualities of the contiguous resident bone. Healing interval, 16 weeks. (*Modified from* Hanisch O, Tatakis DN, Rohrer MD, et al. Bone formation and osseointegration stimulated by rhBMP-2 following subantral augmentation procedures in nonhuman primates. Int J Oral Maxillofac Implants 1997;12:785–92; with permission.)

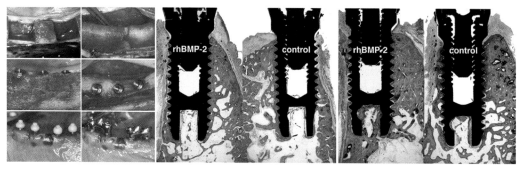

Fig. 7. Evaluation of titanium implants placed into rhBMP-2–induced bone subject to 12 months of functional loading. The clinical panels show surgically induced mandibular, saddle-type (approximately 15 × 10 mm), full-thickness alveolar ridge defects (two per jaw quadrant). The defects were immediately implanted with rhBMP-2/ACS with or without a barrier membrane. Healing progressed for 3 months when endosseous oral implants were installed into the rhBMP-2/ACS–induced bone and into the contiguous resident bone (control). After 4 months of osseointegration, the implants received abutments and prosthetic reconstruction. Prosthetically reconstructed implants were then subject to functional loading for 12 months. The photomicrographs show implants placed into rhBMP-2–induced and resident bone after 12 months of functional loading. There is no discernable difference in bone formation and osseointegration between rhBMP-2–induced and resident bone. (*Modified from* Jovanovic SA, Hunt DR, Bernard GW, et al. Long-term functional loading of dental implants in rhBMP-2 induced bone: a histologic study in the canine ridge augmentation model. Clin Oral Implants Res 2003;14:793–803; with permission.)

[62,63,73] for maxillary sinus augmentation. The reports described three patients receiving the rhOP-1/demineralized bovine bone matrix construct. Control patients received demineralized bovine bone matrix ($n = 3$), autogenous bone grafts ($n = 3$), or served as untreated controls ($n = 3$). Six months upon implantation, sites subject to sinus augmentation showed increased bone formation compared with untreated controls. Sites that received autogenous bone showed lamellar bone formation. Sites that received demineralized bovine bone matrix showed mostly woven bone formation. Sites that received rhOP-1/demineralized bovine bone matrix showed bone formation of varying qualities in two of three patients: one patient showed well-vascularized bone-like tissue, a second patient showed some bone-like formation, and the third patient showed no bone formation. The implanted site exhibited a cyst-like granular tissue without purulent content, however. These observations may indicate that this rhOP-1 construct has a potential to induce bone formation for sinus augmentation; however, considerable variability in treatment outcomes among patients suggests that further development seems necessary before clinical introduction.

A 4-month, open-label, phase I study assessed the safety and technical feasibility of rhBMP-2/ACS for sinus augmentation [60]. This was the first clinical study that evaluated rhBMP-2/ACS for this indication. Twelve patients with inadequate bone height in the posterior maxilla were evaluated. rhBMP-2 dose/patient ranged from 1.8 to 3.4 mg. The rhBMP-2/ACS construct was easily handled. Significant bone growth was documented by CT scans. The overall mean height for the maxillary sinus floor augmentation was 8.5 mm. There were no serious or unexpected immunologic or other adverse effects and no significant changes in blood counts/chemistries or urine analysis. The most frequent adverse effects were facial edema, oral erythema, pain, and rhinitis. Histologic examinations of core biopsies obtained at the time of oral implant installation showed that the rhBMP-2/ACS–induced bone did not significantly differ from the adjoining resident bone and that it was acceptable for placement of endosseous oral implants.

A subsequent phase II study evaluated two concentrations of rhBMP-2 for safety and efficacy in inducing adequate bone formation for placement of endosseous oral implants in patients who required sinus augmentation [61]. Patients received rhBMP-2/ACS (rhBMP-2 at 0.75 and 1.5 mg/mL) or bone graft. rhBMP-2/ACS–induced bone formation was evaluated using CT scans obtained before, at 4 months after treatment, and at 6 months after functional loading of the implants. Mean increase in alveolar ridge height at 4 months approximated 10 mm for the rhBMP-2/ACS groups versus 11 mm for the bone graft group. Core biopsies obtained at implant placement confirmed normal bone formation.

The proportion of patients who received endosseous implants that were functionally loaded and remained functional at 36 months after functional loading was 67% and 76% for the rhBMP-2/ACS 0.75mg/mL and 1.5 mg/mL groups, respectively, versus 62% for the bone graft group. Collectively, these reports suggested that rhBMP-2/ACS seems to be a safe and effective alternative to bone grafts in patients who require maxillary sinus floor augmentation procedures; rhBMP-2/ACS–induced bone assumes qualities of the contiguous maxillary resident bone, which allows placement and long-term functional loading of endosseous oral implants.

Alveolar ridge augmentation

Alveolar ridge augmentation has been evaluated using rhBMP-2/ACS and rhBMP-2 combined with a bovine bone biomaterial [51,54,77,78]. Two reports concerned 12 patients treated with rhBMP-2/ACS used as an inlay in extraction sites and as an onlay for sites that required alveolar ridge augmentation. rhBMP-2 dose/patient ranged from 0.2 to 1.75 mg. Patient safety was monitored using oral examinations, radiographs, and collection of blood samples to assess serum chemistries, hematology, and antibody formation. Radiographic evaluations included bone height, width, and density using CT scans. Short-term results suggested that the rhBMP-2/ACS was well tolerated—locally and systemically—without significant adverse events [51]. The rhBMP-2/ACS was—without difficulty—adapted to extraction sockets and the alveolar ridge. The experimental sites were firm to palpation at week 4; loss of volume was noted for some sites between weeks 4 and 8. All extraction sites exhibited satisfactory bone fill. The alveolar ridge augmentation procedure resulted in limited, clinically irrelevant, increased bone height (mean 0.2 mm). No significant or unexpected adverse events were observed during the 2 years after implantation [77]. Adverse events were mostly benign and compatible with routine oral implant surgeries; ten patients (six extraction socket sites and four ridge augmentation sites) were functionally restored with endosseous oral implants. Histologic evaluation of core biopsies obtained at implant placement showed normal physiologic bone indistinguishable from the resident bone. Clinical examinations revealed that all oral implants exhibited stable marginal bone levels and healthy peri-implant tissues. Importantly, these observations must be viewed in perspective of the lack of controls

in particular for appreciation of the outcomes in extraction sites. As has been observed repeatedly in preclinical models, rhBMP-2/ACS lacks structural integrity for adequate bone formation when used for onlay indications (in this study, alveolar ridge augmentation) so observed negligible effects should be expected [48,49].

A separate study evaluated 80 patients who exhibited extraction socket buccal wall defects ($\geq 50\%$ loss of the buccal wall) at maxillary anterior or premolar teeth immediately after tooth extraction [78]. Two cohorts of 40 patients each were randomized in a double-masked protocol to receive rhBMP-2/ACS (rhBMP-2 at 0.75 and 1.5 mg/mL), ACS alone, and sham control. Efficacy was assessed by evaluating the amount of bone induction (height and width) and adequacy of the alveolar bone to support placement of endosseous implants without need for a secondary augmentation procedure at 4 months after surgery. Extraction sites that received rhBMP-2/ACS using the 1.5 mg/mL concentration exhibited significantly greater bone augmentation than the controls ($P \leq .05$). Adequate bone volume for placement of endosseous implants was observed approximately twice as often compared with controls. Bone density and histology assessments revealed no relevant differences between the newly formed and resident bone. The results from this study demonstrated that rhBMP-2/ACS produces a clinically relevant effect in this rare indication. Clinicians, however, must be aware that these observations may be unique to this limited indication and do not necessarily translate to other onlay/inlay indications in the dentoalveolar complex.

A third study evaluated 11 partially edentulous patients who required alveolar ridge augmentation at two different sites in conjunction with placement of endosseous oral implants using rhBMP-2 coated onto bovine bone particles combined with GBR [54]. Controls received bovine bone particles without rhBMP-2 combined with GBR. Average defect height was 7.0 and 5.8 mm for the rhBMP-2 and control group, respectively. Defect resolution, measured during re-entry surgery at 6 months, amounted to 96% and 91% for the rhBMP-2 and control group, respectively. A histologic/histometric evaluation of core biopsies from the experimental sites revealed bone formation among the bovine bone particles without evidence of resorption of the biomaterial; fraction newly formed bone amounted to 37% and 30% for the rhBMP-2 and control group, respectively. The results did not reveal a remarkable or relevant effect of this rhBMP-2 construct. Clinicians, however, should be concerned about the apparently nonresorbing bone biomaterial used as a carrier technology. Although the implants were stable during the healing sequel, the long-term effects of such biomaterials sequestered in bone are unknown. Do they compromise biomechanical stability of bone and ultimately osseointegration? Do they influence bone remodeling and ultimately osseointegration? Do they accelerate infectious processes associated with peri-implantitis and, ultimately, osseointegration? Observations in preclinical models suggested that nonresorbable or slowly resorbable biomaterials displace rhBMP-2–induced bone formation when used for onlay indications, which results in considerable expansion of the experimental sites and poor bone quality [48,100]. On the other hand, the use of space-providing, rapidly resorbing biomaterials as carrier technologies for rhBMP-2 allows clinically relevant bone formation and osseointegration indistinguishable from that of adjoining resident bone [87].

Overall, the effect of BMP technologies in clinical studies evaluating alveolar augmentation indications seems less promising than that of the maxillary sinus. The innate healing potential of the extraction sites makes this indication a particularly difficult target of study. As has been convincingly demonstrated in preceding preclinical models [48,49,100], the biomaterials chosen as carrier technologies for rhBMP-2— whether being ACS without structural integrity or the nonresorbable or slowly resorbable bone biomaterial—may each in their unique ways contribute to the observed limited or compromised bone formation.

Segmental/resection defects

Craniofacial reconstruction using BMPs, including chronic and acute posttraumatic discontinuity defects, congenital malformations (Apert and Crouzon syndromes), and large (tumor) resection defects have been reported [33,34,45]. A recent report demonstrated the reconstruction of a mandibular resection defect using rhOP-1 in a custom scaffold for human ectopic/heterotopic bone formation [45]. CT and computer-aided designs were used to produce a virtual replacement for the mandibular defect; to design and manufacture a custom titanium mesh cage that was filled with bone mineral blocks and infiltrated with 7 mg rhOP-1 and 20 mL autogenous bone marrow. The rhOP-1 construct was implanted into the

Latissimus dorsi muscle and 7 weeks later transplanted as a free bone-muscle flap to the mandibular site. Skeletal scintigraphy showed bone remodeling and mineralization inside the mandibular transplant before and after transplantation. CT provided radiologic evidence of new bone formation. Upon transplantation, the patient exhibited improved mastication and was satisfied with the aesthetic outcome. This case report demonstrated the significant principle of predetermined scaffolds using ectopic/heterotopic bone induction for craniofacial reconstruction. The application of this principle using orthotopic bone induction for alveolar ridge augmentation has been demonstrated using preclinical models [88,89].

Summary

Preclinical studies have shown that rhBMP-2 induces normal physiologic bone in clinically relevant defects in the craniofacial skeleton. The newly formed bone assumes characteristics of the adjacent resident bone and allows placement, osseointegration/re-osseointegration, and functional loading of endosseous implants. Clinical studies optimizing dose, delivery technologies, and conditions for stimulation of bone growth will bring about a new era in dentistry. The ability to predictably promote osteogenesis through the use of BMP-technologies is not far from becoming a clinical reality and will undoubtedly have an astounding effect on how dentistry is practiced.

References

[1] Li RH, Wozney JM. Delivering on the promise of bone morphogenetic proteins. Trends Biotechnol 2001;19:255–65.

[2] Schilephake H. Bone growth factors in maxillofacial skeletal reconstruction. Int J Oral Maxillofac Surg 2002;31:469–84.

[3] Urist MR. Bone: formation by autoinduction. Science 1965;150:893–9.

[4] Urist MR, Strates BS. Bone morphogenetic protein. J Dent Res 1971;50:S1392–406.

[5] Hötten GC, Matsumoto T, Kimura M, et al. Recombinant human growth/differentiation factor 5 stimulates mesenchyme aggregation and chondrogenesis responsible for the skeletal development of limbs. Growth Factors 1996;13:65–74.

[6] Sampath TK, Maliakal JC, Hauschka PV, et al. Recombinant human osteogenic protein-1 (hOP-1) induces new bone formation in vivo with a specific activity comparable with natural bovine osteogenic

protein and stimulates osteoblast proliferation and differentiation in vitro. J Biol Chem 1992;267: 20352–62.

[7] Wang EA, Rosen V, D'Alessandro JS, et al. Recombinant human bone morphogenetic protein induces bone formation. Proc Natl Acad Sci U S A 1990;87:2220–4.

[8] Celeste AJ, Iannazzi JA, Taylor RC, et al. Identification of transforming growth factor ß family members present in bone-inductive protein purified from bovine bone. Proc Natl Acad Sci U S A 1990; 87:9843–7.

[9] Özkaynak E, Rueger DC, Drier EA, et al. OP-1 cDNA encodes an osteogenic protein in the TGF-ß family. EMBO J 1990;9:2085–93.

[10] Wozney JM, Rosen V, Celeste AJ, et al. Novel regulators of bone formation: molecular clones and activities. Science 1988;242:1528–34.

[11] Urist MR. The substratum for bone morphogenesis. Symp Soc Dev Biol 1970;4:125–63.

[12] Urist MR, Huo YK, Brownell AG, et al. Purification of bovine bone morphogenetic protein by hydroxyapatite chromatography. Proc Natl Acad Sci U S A 1984;81:371–5.

[13] Israel DI, Nove J, Kerns KM, et al. Expression and characterization of bone morphogenetic protein-2 in Chinese hamster ovary cells. Growth Factors 1992;7:139–50.

[14] Zhao M, Wang H, Zhou T. Expression of recombinant mature peptide of human bone morphogenetic protein-2 in Escherichia coli and its activity in bone formation. Chin Biochem J 1994;10: 319–24.

[15] Mikulski AJ, Urist MR. An antigenic antimorphogenic bone hydrophobic glycopeptide (AHG). Prep Biochem 1975;5:21–37.

[16] Tomford W. Transmission of disease through transplantation of musculoskeletal allografts. J Bone Joint Surg Am 1995;77:1742–54.

[17] Boden SD. Clinical application of the BMPs. J Bone Joint Surg Am 2001;83:S161.

[18] Bostrom MP, Camacho NP. Potential role of bone morphogenetic proteins in fracture healing. Clin Orthop Relat Res 1998;355:S274–82.

[19] Cook SD. Preclinical and clinical evaluation of osteogenic protein-1 (BMP-7) in bony sites. Orthopedics 1999;22:669–71.

[20] Cook SD, Barrack RL, Shimmin A, et al. The use of osteogenic protein-1 in reconstructive surgery of the hip. J Arthroplasty 2001;16:88–94.

[21] Friedlaender GE, Perry CR, Cole JD, et al. Osteogenic protein-1 (bone morphogenetic protein-7) in the treatment of tibial nonunions. J Bone Joint Surg Am 2001;83:S151–8.

[22] Friedlaender GE. OP-1 clinical studies. J Bone Joint Surg Am 2001;83:S160–1.

[23] Kuslich SD, Ulstrom CL, Griffith SL, et al. The Bagby and Kuslich method of lumbar interbody fusion: history, techniques, and 2-year follow-up

results of a United States prospective, multicenter trial. Spine 1998;23:1267–79.

[24] McKay B, Sandhu HS. Use of recombinant human bone morphogenetic protein-2 in spinal fusion applications. Spine 2002;27:S66–85.

[25] Spiro RC, Liu L-S, Heidaran MA, et al. Inductive activity of recombinant human growth and differentiation factor-5. Biochem Soc Trans 2000;28:362–8.

[26] Vaccaro AR, Anderson DG, Toth CA. Recombinant human osteogenic protein-1 (bone morphogenetic protein-7) as an osteoinductive agent in spinal fusion. Spine 2002;27:S59–65.

[27] Valentin-Opran A, Wozney J, Csimma C, et al. Clinical evaluation of recombinant human bone morphogenetic protein-2. Clin Orthop Relat Res 2002;395:110–20.

[28] Boyne PJ. Animal studies of the application of rhBMP-2 in maxillofacial reconstruction. Bone 1996;19:S83–92.

[29] Boyne PJ, Nath R, Nakamura A. Human recombinant BMP-2 in osseous reconstruction of simulated cleft palate defects. Br J Oral Maxillofac Surg 1998; 36:84–90.

[30] Boyne PJ, Nakamura A, Shabahang S. Evaluation of the long-term effect of function on rhBMP-2 regenerated hemimandibulectomy defects. Br J Oral Maxillofac Surg 1999;37:344–52.

[31] Marukawa E, Asahina I, Oda M, et al. Functional reconstruction of the non-human primate mandible using recombinant human bone morphogenetic protein-2. Int J Oral Maxillofac Surg 2002;31:287–95.

[32] Mayer M, Hollinger J, Ron E, et al. Maxillary alveolar cleft repair in dogs using recombinant human bone morphogenetic protein-2 and a polymer carrier. Plast Reconstr Surg 1996;98:247–59.

[33] Moghadam HG, Urist MR, Sandor GK, et al. Successful mandibular reconstruction using a BMP bioimplant. J Craniofac Surg 2001;12:119–27 [discussion: 128].

[34] Sailer HF, Kolb E. Application of purified bone morphogenetic protein (BMP) preparations in cranio-maxillo-facial surgery: reconstruction in craniofacial malformations and post-traumatic or operative defects of the skull with lyophilized cartilage and BMP. J Craniomaxillofac Surg 1994;22: 191–9.

[35] Sheehan JP, Sheehan JM, Seeherman H, et al. The safety and utility of recombinant human bone morphogenetic protein-2 for cranial procedures in a nonhuman primate model. J Neurosurg 2003; 98:125–30.

[36] Springer IN, Acil Y, Kuchenbecker S, et al. Bone graft versus BMP-7 in a critical size defect: cranioplasty in a growing infant model. Bone 2005;37: 563–9.

[37] Steinberg B, Chiego DJ Jr, Huizinga PJ, et al. Effect of human bone morphogenetic protein-2 implant on tooth eruption in an experimental design. J Craniofac Surg 1999;10:338–41.

[38] Terheyden H, Jepsen S, Rueger DR. Mandibular reconstruction in miniature pigs with prefabricated vascularized bone grafts using recombinant human osteogenic protein-1: a preliminary study. Int J Oral Maxillofac Surg 1999;28:461–3.

[39] Terheyden H, Knak C, Jepsen S, et al. Mandibular reconstruction with a prefabricated vascularized bone graft using recombinant human osteogenic protein-1: an experimental study in miniature pigs. Part I: prefabrication. Int J Oral Maxillofac Surg 2001;30:373–9.

[40] Terheyden H, Warnke P, Dunsche A, et al. Mandibular reconstruction with prefabricated vascularized bone grafts using recombinant human osteogenic protein-1: an experimental study in miniature pigs. Part II: transplantation. Int J Oral Maxillofac Surg 2001;30:469–78.

[41] Terheyden H, Wang H, Warnke PH, et al. Acceleration of callus maturation using rhOP-1 in mandibular distraction osteogenesis in a rat model. Int J Oral Maxillof Surg 2003;32:528–33.

[42] Terheyden H, Menzel C, Wang H, et al. Prefabrication of vascularized bone grafts using recombinant human osteogenic protein-1. Part 3: dosage of rhOP-1, the use of external and internal scaffolds. Int J Oral Maxillofac Surg 2004;33:164–72.

[43] Toriumi DM, Kotler HS, Luxenberg DP, et al. Mandibular reconstruction with a recombinant bone-inducing factor: functional, histologic, and biomechanical evaluation. Arch Otolaryngol Head Neck Surg 1991;117:1101–12.

[44] Toriumi DM, O'Grady K, Horlbeck DM, et al. Mandibular reconstruction using bone morphogenetic protein 2: long-term follow-up in a canine model. Laryngoscope 1999;109:1481–9.

[45] Warnke PH, Springer IN, Wiltfang J, et al. Growth and transplantation of a custom vascularised bone graft in a man. Lancet 2004;364:766–70.

[46] Warnke PH, Springer IN, Acil Y, et al. The mechanical integrity of in vivo engineered heterotopic bone. Biomaterials 2006;27:1081–7.

[47] Yudell RM, Block MS. Bone gap healing in the dog using recombinant human bone morphogenetic protein-2. J Oral Maxillofac Surg 2000;58:761–6.

[48] Barboza EP, Leite Duarte ME, Geolás L, et al. Ridge augmentation following implantation of recombinant human bone morphogenetic protein-2 in the dog. J Periodontol 2000;71:488–96.

[49] Barboza E, Caúla AL, Caúla F, et al. Effect of recombinant human bone morphogenetic protein-2 in an absorbable collagen sponge with space-providing biomaterials on the augmentation of chronic alveolar ridge defects. J Periodontol 2004; 75:702–8.

[50] Bergenholtz GI, Wikesjö UME, Sorensen RG, et al. Observations on healing following endodontic surgery in nonhuman primates (Macaca fascicularis): effects of rhBMP-2. Oral Surg Oral Med Oral Pathol Oral Radiol Endod 2006;101:116–25.

[51] Howell TH, Fiorellini J, Jones A, et al. A feasibility study evaluating rhBMP-2/absorbable collagen sponge device for local alveolar ridge preservation or augmentation. Int J Periodontics Restorative Dent 1997;17:124–39.

[52] Hunt DR, Jovanovic SA, Wikesjö UME, et al. Hyaluronan supports recombinant human bone morphogenetic protein-2 induced bone reconstruction of advanced alveolar ridge defects in dogs: a pilot study. J Periodontol 2001;72:651–8.

[53] Jovanovic SA, Hunt DR, Bernard GW, et al. Bone reconstruction following implantation of rhBMP-2 and guided bone regeneration in canine alveolar ridge defects. Clin Oral Implants Res 2007;18: 224–30.

[54] Jung RE, Glauser R, Schärer P, et al. Effect of rhBMP-2 on guided bone regeneration in humans. Clin Oral Implants Res 2003;14:556–68.

[55] Marukawa E, Asahina I, Oda M, et al. Bone regeneration using recombinant human bone morphogenetic protein-2 (rhBMP-2) in alveolar defects of primate mandibles. Br J Oral Maxillofac Surg 2001;39:452–9.

[56] Miranda DAO, Blumenthal NM, Sorensen RG, et al. Evaluation of recombinant human bone morphogenetic protein-2 on the repair of alveolar ridge defects in baboons. J Periodontol 2005;76:210–20.

[57] Roldan JC, Jepsen S, Miller J, et al. Bone formation in the presence of platelet-rich plasma vs. bone morphogenetic protein-7. Bone 2004;34:80–90.

[58] Terheyden H, Jepsen S, Vogeler S, et al. Recombinant human osteogenic protein 1 in the rat mandibular augmentation model: differences in morphology of the newly formed bone are dependent on the type of carrier. Mund Kiefer Gesichtschir 1997;1:272–5.

[59] Wikesjö UME, Sorensen RG, Wozney JM. Augmentation of alveolar bone and dental implant osseointegration: clinical implications of studies with rhBMP-2. A comprehensive review. J Bone Joint Surg Am 2001;83:S136–45.

[60] Boyne PJ, Marx RE, Nevins M, et al. A feasibility study evaluating rhBMP-2/absorbable collagen sponge for maxillary sinus floor augmentation. Int J Periodontics Restorative Dent 1997;17:11–25.

[61] Boyne PJ, Lilly LC, Marx RE, et al. De novo bone induction by recombinant human bone morphogenetic protein-2 (rhBMP-2) in maxillary sinus floor augmentation. J Oral Maxillofac Surg 2005;63: 1693–707.

[62] Groeneveld EH, van den Bergh JP, Holzmann P, et al. Histomorphometrical analysis of bone formed in human maxillary sinus floor elevations grafted with OP-1 device, demineralized bone matrix or autogenous bone: comparison with nongrafted sites in a series of case reports. Clin Oral Implants Res 1999;10:499–509.

[63] Groenveld HH, van den Bergh JP, Holzmann P, et al. Histological observations of a bilateral

maxillary sinus floor elevation 6 and 12 months after grafting with osteogenic protein-1 device. J Clin Periodontol 1999;26:841–6.

[64] Hanisch O, Tatakis DN, Rohrer MD, et al. Bone formation and osseointegration stimulated by rhBMP-2 following subantral augmentation procedures in nonhuman primates. Int J Oral Maxillofac Implants 1997;12:785–92.

[65] Kirker-Head CA, Nevins M, Palmer R, et al. A new animal model for maxillary sinus floor augmentation: evaluation parameters. Int J Oral Maxillofac Implants 1997;12:403–11.

[66] Ludwig A, Gruber R, Nitsch A, et al. GDF-5 coated beta-TCP in sinus augmentation in minipigs. Int J Oral Maxillofac Surg 2003;32:S1:55.

[67] Margolin MD, Cogan AG, Taylor M, et al. Maxillary sinus augmentation in the non-human primate: a comparative radiographic and histologic study between recombinant human osteogenic protein-1 and natural bone mineral. J Periodontol 1998;69:911–9.

[68] McAllister BS, Margolin MD, Cogan AG, et al. Residual lateral wall defects following sinus grafting with recombinant human osteogenic protein-1 or Bio-Oss in the chimpanzee. Int J Periodontics Restorative Dent 1998;18:227–39.

[69] Nevins M, Kirker-Head CA, Nevins M, et al. Bone formation in the goat maxillary sinus induced by absorbable collagen sponge implants impregnated with recombinant human bone morphogenetic protein-2. Int J Periodontics Restorative Dent 1996;16: 8–19.

[70] Roldan JC, Jepsen S, Schmidt C, et al. Sinus floor augmentation with simultaneous placement of dental implants in the presence of platelet-rich plasma or recombinant human bone morphogenetic protein-7. Clin Oral Implants Res 2004;15:716–23.

[71] Terheyden H, Jepsen S, Möller B, et al. Sinus floor augmentation with simultaneous placement of dental implants using a combination of deproteinized bone xenografts and recombinant human osteogenic protein-1: a histometric study in miniature pigs. Clin Oral Implants Res 1999;10:510–21.

[72] Terheyden H, Jepsen S, Möller B, et al. [Sinus floor augmentation with simultaneous implant insertion using recombinant human osteogenic protein-1]. Laryngorhinootologie 2001;80:47–51 [in German].

[73] van den Bergh JP, ten Bruggenkate CM, Groeneveld HH, et al. Recombinant human bone morphogenetic protein-7 in maxillary sinus floor elevation surgery in 3 patients compared to autogenous bone grafts: A clinical pilot study. J Clin Periodontol 2000;27:627–36.

[74] Boyne PJ, Shabahang S. An evaluation of bone induction delivery materials in conjunction with root-form implant placement. Int J Periodontics Restorative Dent 2001;21:333–43.

[75] Cochran DL, Nummikoski PV, Jones AA, et al. Radiographic analysis of regenerated bone around endosseous implants in canine using recombinant

human bone morphogenetic protein-2. Int J Oral Maxillofac Implants 1997;12:739–48.

[76] Cochran DL, Schenk R, Buser D, et al. Recombinant human bone morphogenetic protein-2 stimulation of bone formation around endosseous dental implants. J Periodontol 1999;70:139–51.

[77] Cochran DL, Jones AA, Lilly LC, et al. Evaluation of recombinant human bone morphogenetic protein-2 in oral applications including the use of endosseous implants: 3-year results of a pilot study in humans. J Periodontol 2000;71:1241–57.

[78] Fiorellini JP, Howell TH, Cochran D, et al. Randomized study evaluating recombinant human bone morphogenetic protein-2 for extraction socket augmentation. J Periodontol 2005;76:605–13.

[79] Hanisch O, Tatakis DN, Boskovic MM, et al. Bone formation and reosseointegration in peri-implantitis defects following surgical implantation of rhBMP-2. Int J Oral Maxillofac Implants 1997; 12:604–10.

[80] Hanisch O, Sorensen RG, Kinoshita A, et al. Effect of recombinant human bone morphogenetic protein-2 in dehiscence defects with non-submerged immediate implants: an experimental study in Cynomolgus monkeys. J Periodontol 2003;74:648–57.

[81] Jovanovic SA, Hunt DR, Bernard GW, et al. Long-term functional loading of dental implants in rhBMP-2 induced bone: a histologic study in the canine ridge augmentation model. Clin Oral Implants Res 2003;14:793–803.

[82] Seto I, Tachikawa N, Mori M, et al. Restoration of occlusal function using osseointegrated implants in the canine mandible reconstructed by rhBMP-2. Clin Oral Implants Res 2002;13: 536–41.

[83] Sigurdsson TJ, Fu E, Tatakis DN, et al. Bone morphogenetic protein-2 enhances peri-implant bone regeneration and osseointegration. Clin Oral Implants Res 1997;8:367–74.

[84] Sigurdsson TJ, Nguyen S, Wikesjö UME. Alveolar ridge augmentation with rhBMP-2 and bone to implant contact in induced bone. Int J Periodontics Restorative Dent 2001;21:461–73.

[85] Sykaras N, Triplett RG, Nunn ME, et al. Effect of recombinant human bone morphogenetic protein-2 on bone regeneration and osseointegration of dental implants. Clin Oral Implants Res 2001;12: 339–49.

[86] Tatakis DN, Koh A, Jin L, et al. Peri-implant bone regeneration using rhBMP-2/ACS in a canine model: a dose-response study. J Periodontal Res 2002;37:93–100.

[87] Wikesjö UME, Sorensen RG, Kinoshita A, et al. rhBMP-2/α-BSM® induces significant vertical alveolar ridge augmentation and dental implant osseointegration. Clin Implant Dent Relat Res 2002;4:173–81.

[88] Wikesjö UME, Qahash M, Thomson RC, et al. Space-providing expanded polytetrafluoroethylene

devices define alveolar augmentation at dental implants induced by recombinant human bone morphogenetic protein-2. Clin Implant Dent Relat Res 2003;5:112–23.

[89] Wikesjö UME, Qahash M, Thomson RC, et al. rhBMP-2 significantly enhances guided bone regeneration. Clin Oral Implants Res 2004;15:194–204.

[90] Blumenthal NM, Koh-Kunts G, Alves MEAF, et al. Effect of surgical implantation of recombinant human bone morphogenetic protein-2 in a bioabsorbable collagen sponge or a calcium phosphate putty carrier in intrabony periodontal defects in the baboon. J Periodontol 2002;73:1494–506.

[91] Choi S-H, Kim C-K, Cho K-S, et al. Effect of recombinant human bone morphogenetic protein-2/absorbable collagen sponge (rhBMP-2/ACS) on healing in 3-wall intrabony defects in dogs. J Periodontol 2002;73:63–72.

[92] Giannobile WV, Ryan S, Shih M-S, et al. Recombinant human osteogenic protein-1 (OP-1) stimulates periodontal wound healing in class III furcation defects. J Periodontol 1998;69:129–37.

[93] Ishikawa I, Kinoshita A, Oda S, et al. Regenerative therapy in periodontal disease: histological observations after implantation of rhBMP-2 in the surgically created periodontal defects in adults dogs. Dent Jpn 1994;31:141–6.

[94] Kinoshita A, Oda S, Takahashi K, et al. Periodontal regeneration by application of recombinant human bone morphogenetic protein-2 to horizontal circumferential defects created by experimental periodontitis in beagle dogs. J Periodontol 1997; 68:103–9.

[95] Ripamonti U, Heliotis M, Rueger DC, et al. Induction of cementogenesis by recombinant human osteogenic protein-1 (hop-1/bmp-7) in the baboon (*Papio ursinus*): short communication. Arch Oral Biol 1996;41:121–6.

[96] Saito E, Saito A, Kawanami M. Favorable healing following space creation in rhBMP-2-induced periodontal regeneration of horizontal circumferential defects in dogs with experimental periodontitis. J Periodontol 2003;74:1808–15.

[97] Selvig KA, Sorensen RG, Wozney JM, et al. Bone repair following recombinant human bone morphogenetic protein-2 stimulated periodontal regeneration. J Periodontol 2002;73:1020–9.

[98] Sigurdsson TJ, Lee MB, Kubota K, et al. Periodontal repair in dogs: recombinant human bone morphogenetic protein-2 significantly enhances periodontal regeneration. J Periodontol 1995;66: 131–8.

[99] Sigurdsson TJ, Tatakis DN, Lee MB, et al. Periodontal regenerative potential of space-providing expanded polytetrafluoroethylene membranes and recombinant human bone morphogenetic proteins. J Periodontol 1995;66:511–21.

[100] Sigurdsson TJ, Nygaard L, Tatakis DN, et al. Periodontal repair in dogs: evaluation of rhBMP-2

carriers. Int J Periodontics Restorative Dent 1996; 16:524–37.

[101] Sorensen RG, Polimeni G, Kinoshita A, et al. Effect of recombinant human bone morphogenetic protein-12 (rhBMP-12) on regeneration of periodontal attachment following tooth replantation in dogs: a pilot study. J Clin Periodontol 2004;31: 654–61.

[102] Sorensen RG, Wikesjö UME, Kinoshita A, et al. Periodontal repair in dogs: evaluation of a bioresorbable calcium phosphate cement (Ceredex™) as a carrier for rhBMP-2. J Clin Periodontol 2004;31:796–804.

[103] Springer IN, Acil Y, Spies C, et al. rhBMP-7 improves survival and eruption in a growing tooth avulsion trauma model. Bone 2005;37:570–7.

[104] Wikesjö UME, Guglielmoni PG, Promsudthi A, et al. Periodontal repair in dogs: effect of rhBMP-2 concentration on regeneration of alveolar bone and periodontal attachment. J Clin Periodontol 1999; 26:392–400.

[105] Wikesjö UME, Lim WH, Thomson RC, et al. Periodontal repair in dogs: evaluation of a bioresorbable space-providing macro-porous membrane with recombinant human bone morphogenetic protein-2. J Periodontol 2003;74:635–47.

[106] Wikesjö UME, Xiropaidis AV, Thomson RC, et al. Periodontal repair in dogs: rhBMP-2 significantly enhances bone formation under provisions for guided tissue regeneration. J Clin Periodontol 2003;30:705–14.

[107] Wikesjö UME, Xiropaidis AV, Thomson RC, et al. Periodontal repair in dogs: space-providing ePTFE devices increase rhBMP-2/ACS induced bone formation. J Clin Periodontol 2003;30:715–25.

[108] Wikesjö UME, Sorensen RG, Kinoshita A, et al. Periodontal repair in dogs: effect of recombinant human bone morphogenetic protein-12 (rhBMP-12) on regeneration of alveolar bone and periodontal attachment. J Clin Periodontol 2004;31: 662–70.

[109] Yamazaki Y, Oida S, Akimoto Y, et al. Response of the mouse femoral muscle to an implant of a composite of bone morphogenetic protein and plaster of Paris. Clin Orthop Relat Res 1988;234: 240–9.

[110] Cole BJ, Bostrom MP, Pritchard TL, et al. Use of bone morphogenetic protein 2 on ectopic porous coated implants in the rat. Clin Orthop Relat Res 1997;345:219–28.

[111] Esenwein SA, Esenwein S, Herr G, et al. [Osteogenetic activity of BMP-3-coated titanium specimens of different surface texture at the orthotopic implant bed of giant rabbits]. Chirurg 2001;72: 1360–8 [in German].

[112] Hartwig C-H, Esenwein SA, Pfund A, et al. [Improved osseointegration of titanium implants of different surface characteristics by the use of bone morphogenetic protein (BMP-3): an animal study

performed at the metaphyseal bone bed in dogs]. Z Orthop Ihre Grenzgeb 2003;141:705–11 [in German].

[113] Herr G, Hartwig C-H, Boll C, et al. Ectopic bone formation by composites of BMP and metal implants in rats. Acta Orthop Scand 1996;67:606–10.

[114] Kawai T, Mieki A, Ohno Y, et al. Osteoinductive activity of composites of bone morphogenetic protein and pure titanium. Clin Orthop Relat Res 1993;290:296–305.

[115] Schmidmaier G, Wildemann B, Cromme F, et al. Bone morphogenetic protein-2 coating of titanium implants increases biomechanical strength and accelerates bone remodeling in fracture treatment: a biomechanical and histological study in rats. Bone 2002;30:816–22.

[116] Vehof JW, Mahmood J, Takita H, et al. Ectopic bone formation in titanium mesh loaded with bone morphogenetic protein and coated with calcium phosphate. Plast Reconstr Surg 2001;108:434–43.

[117] Hall J, Sorensen RG, Wozney JM, et al. Bone formation at rhBMP-2-coated titanium implants in the rat ectopic model. J Clin Periodontol 2007;34:444–51.

[118] Jin QM, Anusaksathien O, Webb SA, et al. Gene therapy of bone morphogenetic protein for periodontal tissue engineering. J Periodontol 2003;74: 202–13.

[119] Wikesjö UME, Susin C, Qahash M, et al. The critical-size supraalveolar peri-implant defect model: characteristics and use. J Clin Periodontol 2006; 33:846–54.

[120] Caplanis N, Sigurdsson TJ, Rohrer MD, et al. Effect of allogeneic, freeze-dried, demineralized bone matrix on guided bone regeneration in supra-alveolar peri-implant defects in dogs. Int J Oral Maxillofac Implants 1997;12:634–42.

ELSEVIER
SAUNDERS

Oral Maxillofacial Surg Clin N Am 19 (2007) 553–563

**ORAL AND
MAXILLOFACIAL
SURGERY CLINICS**
of North America

Advances in Head and Neck Radiotherapy to the Mandible

Henry W. Ferguson, DMD*, Mark R. Stevens, DDS

Oral and Maxillofacial Surgery, The Medical College of Georgia, AD 1206, Augusta, GA 30912, USA

Management of radiation-exposed bone in the mandible is a dilemma many oral and maxillofacial surgeons must confront and manage. The mandible resides in an anatomically complex area. It is also co-located in close proximity to anatomic regions that have served historically and frequently as primary sites for head and neck malignancy. In the war against head and neck malignancy and with the use of radiotherapy, a primary weapon in its eradication, the mandible frequently has been a casualty of war. Current advances in radiotherapy techniques using pinpoint computerized accuracy in combination with other advances, such as morphed imaging, fractionalization protocols, minimization of scatter, and pretreatment dental examinations, have greatly decreased the late effects of radiation and osteoradionecrosis (ORN). The intent of this article is to provide a brief overview of the following topics: radiotherapy physics and radiobiology, effects of radiotherapy on normal tissues, including the pathogenesis of ORN, and advances in contemporary radiotherapy treatment.

The use of radiotherapy is a proven therapeutic modality for treatment and palliation of head and neck malignancy [1]. The theory behind its use is that therapeutic radiotherapy targets neoplastic cells because of their innate higher level of cellular turnover. Many normal cell lines also demonstrate high cell turnover rates; those cell lines are also prone to significant radiation injury indicative of the acute and or late effects of radiation. Germinal cells and lymphoreticular cells demonstrate the most sensitivity. Endothelial cells and fibroblasts demonstrate intermediate sensitivity. Muscle and nerve cells demonstrate the least. Endothelial cells and fibroblasts with intermediate sensitivity are some of the most important cell lines to clinicians because of their significant role in the process of healing [2].

Types of radiation used to treat cancer

Radiation used for cancer treatment is called ionizing radiation. It forms ions as it passes through tissues and dislodges electrons from atoms. Ions are atoms that have acquired an electric charge through the gain or loss of an electron. Ionization causes cell death or a genetic change. Other forms of radiation, such as radiowaves, microwaves, and light waves, are called nonionizing and have little energy. Ionizing radiation can be divided into two major types: (1) photons (x-rays and gamma rays) and (2) particle radiation (electrons, protons, neutrons, alpha particles, and beta particles). Some types of ionizing radiation have more energy than others. The higher the energy, the more deeply the radiation can penetrate into the tissues. The way a certain type of radiation behaves is important in planning radiation treatments.

Radiation oncologists select the type and energy of radiation that is most suitable for each patient's cancer. The more common types of radiation used for cancer treatment are as follows:

- High-energy photons come from radioactive sources such as cobalt, cesium, or a linear accelerator.

---
* Corresponding author.
E-mail address: hferguson@mcg.edu
(H.W. Ferguson).

1042-3699/07/$ - see front matter © 2007 Elsevier Inc. All rights reserved.
doi:10.1016/j.coms.2007.07.005

- Electron beams produced by a linear accelerator are used for tumors close to a body surface, and their penetration is minimal.
- Protons are a newer form of treatment. Protons cause little damage to tissues they pass through but are effective at killing cells at the end of their path. Proton beam radiation can deliver more radiation to the tumor while reducing side effects of nearby normal tissues. Unfortunately, proton beam radiation therapy requires highly specialized equipment and is currently only available in a few medical centers.
- Neutrons are used for some cancers of the head, neck, and prostate. Sometimes they can be effective when other forms of radiation therapy are infective. Their use has declined over the years because of severe long-term side effects.

Radiation physics

The goal of radiation therapy is to eradicate a tumor with minimal adverse effects on surrounding normal tissues. To limit the adverse effects on normal tissue, upper limits of the radiation dose and the dose rate that can be used have been identified. The two categories of ionizing radiation are important with reference to their biologic effects: electromagnetic radiation and particulate radiation. Electromagnetic radiation is thought of as existing in packages of energy called photons. If these photons have their origin within the atomic nucleus, they are called gamma rays. If they originate from the electron shell around the atomic nucleus of the radiation source, they are called x-rays. Particulate radiation of importance in radiotherapy includes electrons, photons, alpha particles, neutrons, and heavy charged ions.

The quantity of radiation delivered to a defined area is the radiation dose. The time rate at which the dose is administered is the dose rate. Historically, the units commonly used as a measure of radiation dose included the roentgen and the rad. The roentgen is defined as a unit of exposure dose for x-rays and gamma rays that produces in 1 cm^3 of dry air at standard temperature and pressure ions carrying one electrostatic unit of electricity of either sign. The rad is defined as a unit of absorbed dose and is the amount of radiation of any type that results in the deposition of 100 ergs of energy per gram of tissue. When

calculating the total doses of radiation, familiarity with conversion of units is essential. The United States is one of the only countries that still uses it as a measurement. The preferred unit is the gray. One rad = 0.01 Gy = 0.01 J of energy absorbed per kilogram of matter. One gray is equivalent to 100 rads. Because grays are such large amounts of radiation, medical use of radiation is typically measured in milligrays (mGy). The normal amount of radiation (mGy) in an abdominal radiograph is 1.4 (mGy). In contrast to radiation dosing in radiation therapy, higher doses are used and the centigray (cGy) is used.

Only charged particle radiation is ionizing in tissues. Charged particles transfer energy by disrupting the atomic orbital electron structure of atoms within the tissues. These atoms may be within vital cellular components such as DNA, RNA, enzymes, components of cell walls, or other critical molecules. They also may interact with the numerous water molecules creating free radicals, which further disrupt other cellular molecules. Indirectly, ionizing radiation (eg, neutrons) transfers energy by colliding with nuclei of tissue atoms, which in turn give off directly ionizing charged particles from their nucleus. This energy as x-rays and gamma rays are in turn absorbed by other tissue atoms, which further give off directly ionizing orbital electrons [3].

Radiobiology

Radiation therapy is for the treatment of cancer using ionizing radiation. An important characteristic in ionizing radiation is that it releases sufficient energy to break chemical bonds in a localized area. Ionizing radiation deposits its energy in biologic material through the production of fast charged particles. If the primary energy is an x-ray, gamma ray, or electron, the secondary particles are electrons. Secondary particles are the particles that are ultimately responsible for inflicting biologic injury. Secondary particles produce multiple free radicals responsible for breaking chemical bonds. R reactive particles disrupt three important cellular molecules known to be radiosensitive: nucleic acids, proteins, and lipids.

To provide local tumor control with radiotherapy, in theory the treatment must be able to eradicate every viable cancer cell. A viable cell is one that is capable of unlimited division. Conversely, a nonviable cell is one that is unable to proliferate indefinitely [4]. It is not necessary that the cells be lysed or morphologically altered to be killed. Cell death from irradiation is caused by irreparable damage to DNA and loss of its reproductive nature, although other cellular targets, such as cell membrane, RNA, and enzyme systems, also may be involved. The damage may occur when a secondary electron that results from absorption of an x-ray interacts directly with the critical target or indirectly when a secondary electron interacts with a molecule in the vicinity of the target producing free radicals. In either example, the injury is inflicted close to where the radiate energy is deposited [4].

The deposition of radiant energy is a random event, as is the infliction of radiochemical injury to the target volume. This implies that every cell in the target volume has the same chance of being hit by a given dose of radiotherapy. A given dose of radiotherapy kills the same population of cells in the tumor, not the same number. It takes the same amount of radiation to reduce the tumor cell population from 100 cells to 10 cells as it does to reduce the tumor population from 10 billion cells to 1 billion cells. This principle demonstrates an important implication for radiotherapy. It shows that the amount of radiation needed to eradicate a target volume depends on the total number of viable cells. A greater dose is needed to control a 4-cm tumor than a 1-cm tumor [4,5].

When a secondary electron passes through matter, clusters of dense ionization are distributed along an otherwise sparsely ionizing tract. If a cluster of dense ionization hits a sensitive target cell, it can inflict irreparable damage. If the target cell is hit by an area of sparse ionization, injury may be inflicted that is not sufficient to kill the cell. In the latter case, additional hits are needed for cells receiving sublethal injury, and these cells can be repaired if no further injury occurs. In most tissue, sublethal injury is repaired in as little as 3 hours, although it can take as long as 24 hours [5].

The ability of a cell to repair sublethal injury between fractions has great clinical importance. The biologic effect of this irradiation depends on this fractionation. The greater the number of fractions, the greater the opportunity for cellular repair between the dose fractions and the greater the total dose required to produce cellular death. This becomes important when comparing the normal cell population in the area of a tumor with the tumor cells. The normal cells and tissues are said to demonstrate late injury and the tumor cells to demonstrate acute radiation injury. The concept of fractionation in radiotherapy is important, especially in the head and neck. It allows normal tissue in the radiation field, which provides an opportunity to repair between fractions and minimizes the late effects of radiation, such as ORN. For tumors with greater capability of repair (sublethal radiation injury), radiotherapy may be directed to provide fewer but larger fractions (hypofractionization) to minimize the opportunity of repair between fractions.

The presence of oxygen at the time of radiation therapy significantly enhances the effects of ionizing radiation on living tissues [6]. In most biologic systems, the dose of radiation necessary to kill hypoxic cells is 2.5- to 3-fold greater than that required to kill well-oxygenated ones. Normal tissues are usually well oxygenated; however, tumors often contain hypoxic regions [7]. Because of tumor growth characteristics, capillaries may collapse or be compressed, which limits blood flow and oxygenation to the tumor. Tumors also outgrow their blood supplies [8]. During fractionation tumor cells are depleted. This reduction in total tumor cell numbers diminishes the requirement for oxygen, which allows for compressed or collapsed capillary beds to open for improved blood flow. Chronic hypoxic tumor cells in closer proximity to capillaries that are also well oxygenated are eradicated. This phenomenon of reoxygenation is a primary reason for delivering radiation therapy in a fractionated course over an extended period of time.

Another factor that influences the radiosensitivity of the cell is its position in the cell cycle [3,5,6]. The cell cycle is divided into four stages and can be thought of as beginning in the mitosis stage when the cell is formed as one of a pair of daughter cells. This stage is followed by the G_1 stage, when the cell is occupied by the metabolic activities for which it is specialized. For cells that rarely—if ever—divide, the G_1 stage is termed G_0, and the cell remains in this stage indefinitely. If the cell is programmed to divide, it enters the S stage after the G_1. During the S stage, DNA is synthesized until at the end of S, the amount of DNA has doubled. After the S stage, the dividing cell enters the G_2 phase, a short phase in which the cell occupies its time with metabolic processes other than DNA synthesis, which prepares it for actual cell division. Finally, the cell enters the mitosis stage again, and two new daughter cells are formed, beginning a new cycle.

The radiosensitivity of the cell depends on the stage of the cell cycle. Populations of cells in mixed stages have multiple radiation responses. In general, cell sensitivity to radiotherapy is greatest during the following cycles: G_2, late G_1, early S, and mitosis stages. Relative resistance is seen during the early G_1 and rises to a maximum in late S cycle.

Cell death after radiotherapy can be divided into two classes: interphase death and reproductive death. Interphase death is seen after higher doses of radiation and is not restricted to proliferating cells. It is an important type of death in cells that reproduce less actively. Much of the late effects of radiotherapy in normal tissue arise during the interphase death. Reproductive death is seen only in cells undergoing rapid cell division. This type of cell death results from cell injury leading to faulty mitosis and death within mitosis. This reproductive death can occur over many months or even years. Some cells that die a reproductive death are capable of completing several cell divisions before they die. Others that have lost their capacity for sustained proliferation and are considered reproductively dead continue to be viable but are functionally incapacitated. Reproductive cell death generally occurs at doses of radiotherapy significantly lower than those necessary to produce interphase death. This issue is important to radiotherapists because it helps separate tumor injury from injury to normal tissue. It is also the mechanism underlying the general principle that a more rapidly a cell line is dividing, the more sensitive it is to radiotherapy.

During the S phase cells are undergoing DNA synthesis and they are much more radioresistant than cells in other phases of the cell cycle. This rationale supports fractionation versus large single dose in controlling tumor growth. By fractionation of treatments, cells that survive each treatment redistribute themselves into more sensitive phases, which makes them more susceptible to future fractions. The greater the number of fraction treatments, the greater probability of cells falling into radiation-sensitive phases. The sensitizing effects of redistribution tend to offset the protective effects of fractionation and sublethal damage repair. Redistribution is greatest for cells that are rapidly cycling, which presents cells with greater opportunity to redistribute between those fractionations.

Cells responsible for acute reactions have rapid cycles (eg, skin, mucosa); cells responsible for late effects (eg, connective tissue, brain, muscle,

vascular tissues) demonstrate a slower cycle rate. The net effect of these differences is that tissues responsible for late complications (eg, ORN) are spared more by fractionation than tissues responsible for acute radiation reactions (eg, mucositis).

Tumors are proliferating tissues. It is not advisable to protract the course of radiotherapy. Tumor cell population reduced via surgery should undergo radiotherapy early to minimize reproliferation. Repopulation is a problematic event with rapidly proliferating tumors. The concern for repopulation phenomenon may accelerate treatment schedules that require twice-daily fractionation protocols. After surgical resection, a period of no longer than 4 to 6 weeks should elapse before initiation of postoperative radiation therapy. Radiosensitivity of a tumor was once thought to be related to tumor histology and location [5,9]. Subsequently, the radiosensitivity was related more to the inability to deliver adequate doses of radiation to specific anatomic areas.

Two biologic factors that determine the probability of local control by radiation are the numbers of malignant cells and the proportion of hypoxic cells. Both factors are principally related to the size of the cancer. Large tumors have more malignant cells and a significantly greater proportion of cells existing in a hypoxic state. Head and neck cancers may be described as exophytic, infiltrative, or ulcerative [9]. These characteristics are useful for predicting the response of radiotherapy. In general, well-vascularized exophytic tumors respond well to radiation. Infiltrative and ulcerative lesions are more radioresistant. The latter tumors are frequently more extensive than is apparent clinically and have large hypoxic components.

Because irreparably injured and surviving cells are morphologically indistinguishable, biopsies are of little value in the early postirradiation period. For head and neck cancers, a positive biopsy result is usually not a reliable indicator of persistent disease until approximately 3 months after treatment.

Effects of radiotherapy on normal tissues

The goal of radiation therapy is to eradicate the tumor with minimal adverse effects on normal surrounding tissue. The price a patient pays is the acceptance of a certain degree of normal tissue injury for control of the lethal tumor [3]. Salivary glands and bone are relatively radioresistant, but because of the intense vascular compromise they demonstrate the late effects of radiation. The effects of radiotherapy are classified as acute or late. Acute effects generally subside several weeks after completion of treatment and are not a major problem. Late effects are a major concern because the tissue injury is progressive and permanent. The late effects of radiotherapy for head and neck cancers include damage to the salivary glands with resultant xerostomia, damage to the dentition, mucosal and muscular fibrosis, soft tissue ulceration and necrosis, ORN, cartilage necrosis, and damage to the eye, ear, and central nervous system.

Xerostomia usually occurs when salivary glands are irradiated with doses that exceed 35 cGy (3500 rad) in 3 to 4 weeks. Smaller doses also may have significant effects in salivary gland function. Salivary epithelium has a slow turnover rate. As such, it might be expected that this salivary gland tissue might have a degree of radioresistance. Because of decreased perfusion over time and resultant destruction of the salivary tissue microvasculature, however, the glands become irreparably damaged, which results in glandular atrophy, fibrosis, and degeneration.

Damage to the dentition is seen within and outside of the radiation field. Damage to the entire dentition and associated soft tissues is usually the result of diminished salivary flow and decreased exposure to the protective effects of saliva on the oral hard and soft tissues. With decreased or absent salivary flow and associated enzyme and immunologic absence that opposes the proliferation of carcinogenic bacteria, the dentition is affected. Radiation exposure of the dentition within the field causes pulpal necrosis and odontoblast death (Fig. 1), which results in deterioration of the dentin and the dentino-enamel junction with eventual loss of enamel, and exposure of dentin (Fig. 2) [2]. Teeth inside and outside the radiation fields are involved in these processes. This direct and indirect radiation affect to the dentition and subsequent potential for patients to develop rampant caries predispose patients to severe infections of the jaw, functional limitations, and decreased quality-of-life issues [10].

The initial effects of radiotherapy on the mucosa are seen within the first 1 to 3 weeks after therapy. The mucosa demonstrates an erythematous presentation that progresses to a severe mucositis with or without ulceration. Pain and dysphagia follow, making oral intake of adequate

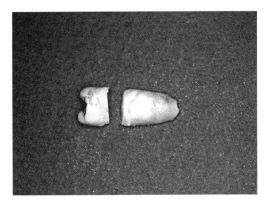

Fig. 1. Postextraction appearance of a tooth in the line of radiation.

nutrition difficult. The acute mucosal reactions subside after completion of the course of radiotherapy. The late effects of radiotherapy involve soft tissue necrosis, ulceration, and delays in healing, even after minor insult. Soft tissue necrosis and ulceration are thought to be the results of radiation damage to vascular connective tissue with disruption of the microvasculature. The mucosa is thinned, less keratinized, and prone to submucosal fibrosis, which makes the oral mucosa less pliable and resilient. The ulcerations may take weeks or months to heal [10].

Dysphagia is one of the most troubling and least treatable complications of radiotherapy. Radiation-induced fibrosis of the pharyngeal constrictors results in lack of coordination necessary to propel a food bolus into the esophagus. This problem results in the common complaint of

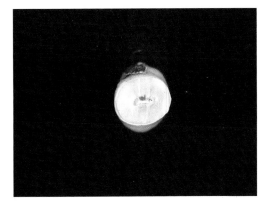

Fig. 2. Cross-section of a radiated tooth demonstrates the chalky desiccated appearance of the dentin and severely narrowed pulpal canal.

difficulty in swallowing and associated higher incidence of aspiration. Radiation fibrosis also extends to the muscles of mastication. Significant fibrosis and trismus within the pterygomasseteric sling cause progressive mandibular hypomobility. Treatment is difficult. Benefits can be gained from bilateral coronoidectomies, but more aggressive attempts to address or remove fibrosed muscle may interfere further with blood supply to the mandibular ramus and increase the predisposition to ORN. In any event, aggressive physiotherapy with jaw-opening exercises and appliances/aids must be used during and after radiotherapy [2].

Osteoradionecrosis

ORN is a debilitating complication of cancer-icidal radiation that involves the osseous structures within the radiation zone [11]. The bone exposed from the radiotherapy becomes virtually nonvital from an endarteritis that results in elimination of fine vascular networks within the bone and decreased perfusion over time. The turnover rate of the remaining viable bone is retarded to the point of having decreased ability for self-repairs. This process of remodeling is essential for normal physiology and daily maintenance of bone. Failure in remodeling of sharp and irregular alveolar surfaces even over considerable periods of time promotes bone exposure. Because the mandible has a greater cortical component, it relies on its blood supply from an endosteal source in contrast to the maxilla. This factor results in the mandible's inability to heal after minor overlying mucosal trauma, which predisposes it to developing osteonecrosis [10].

Initially, ORN was thought to be a radiation-induced osteomyelitis [12]. It was thought that the introduction of sepsis into avascular bone produced a virulent form of osteomyelitis with accompanied soft tissue destruction [13]. Over time with significant investigation and study of ORN, the true pathogenesis sequencing was delineated. The current espoused pathogenesis is exposure of the bone to radiation, development of hypovas-cular-hypocellular tissue, and tissue breakdown (ie, cellular death and collagen lysis that exceed cellular replication and collagen synthesis) followed by a nonhealing wound (eg, tooth extraction), in which oxygen and metabolic demand exceed supply (Fig. 3) [11]. This sequencing best predicts the observation of nonhealing bone with overlying soft tissue breakdown that fails to

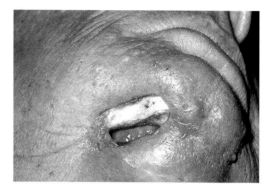

Fig. 3. ORN of the mandible shows nonvital bone and associated oral cutaneous fistula.

resolve despite aggressive wound care, antibiotic therapy, and superficial sequestration. Research and investigation support the premise that antibiotics, which were the mainstay in the treatment and prevention of ORN, are of little therapeutic value in reducing the incidence of ORN [14].

The risk of developing ORN depends on several key factors, including primary site, T staging, proximity of the tumor to bone, condition of the dentition, type of treatment (eg, external beam radiotherapy, brachytherapy, surgery or chemotherapy), and radiotherapy dose. Other factors that influence the likelihood of developing ORN include the nutritional status of the patient and continued use of tobacco products or alcohol abuse.

The mandible is the most common site of ORN in the head. The rationale for this is its proximity to common malignancies, blood supply, cortical composition, and thin overlying mucosa. Patients in whom radiotherapy portals include only the angle or ramus of the mandible, such as persons who have pharyngeal or laryngeal cancers, have a lower likelihood of ORN. Edentulous patients also have a lower risk of developing ORN than dentate patients. Patients with poor dentition whose teeth are in the radiation field have the highest risk for developing ORN. Patients with posterior teeth in the direct line of radiation should undergo extractions before radiotherapy. A period of at least 2 to 3 weeks should elapse before initiating radiotherapy. Whether it is recommended to extract healthy teeth that receive high-dose radiotherapy outside the direct portal is still a topic of controversy. The use of ill-fitting dentures after radiotherapy also can increase the risk of ORN. It is probably best not to use lower dentures after high-dose radiation of 60 cGy (6000 rad) or more.

Advances in radiotherapy

There have been several major technical advances in radiotherapy designed to aggressively address tumor mass while rendering as little collateral radiation injury to uninvolved normal tissues. The positron emission tomography scan has led to improved localization of tumors relative to proximal normal tissues within the complex anatomic confines of the head and neck (Figs. 4 and 5) [15]. Development of advanced computer-generated, three-dimensional reconstructions of correlated CT and MRI has paralleled the advances in imaging, facilitating appreciation of radiation dosimetry from any viewing perspective. Target volumes and critical normal tissues can be identified with greater accuracy in relation to the anatomy of the patient in the treatment position. Patient anatomy can be reconstructed in three dimensions, which provides better diagnostic

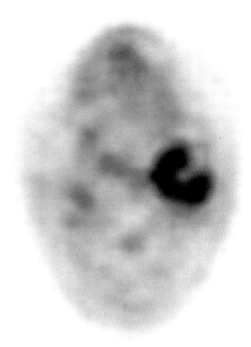

Fig. 5. Neck positron emission tomography scan of the same metastatic squamous cell carcinoma. Scan is used to help delineate disease for precision dose radiation treatment.

information concerning the tumor extensions and relationships with proximal normal tissues. It also has led the way to development of three-dimensional treatment planning. In combining technologic advances, it has been possible to incorporate information from other diagnostic imaging tools (eg, MRI, single photon emission computer tomography, and positron emission tomography) into treatment planning. Incorporation of sophisticated computer software and hardware has increased accuracy of patient positioning for stereotactic radiotherapy treatment (Fig. 6).

Paralleling these improvements have been radical changes in the fractionation patterns (hyperfractionation, accelerated fractionation) and the use of concomitant chemotherapy. Hyperfractionation aims to spare normal tissues relative to the tumor by giving a high total dose spread over a large number of small doses per fraction. Smaller dose per fraction allows normal tissues to repair the radiation-induced damage relatively more efficiently than tumor cells [16]. Randomized clinical trials have demonstrated improved local control rates in head and neck cancer [17,18].

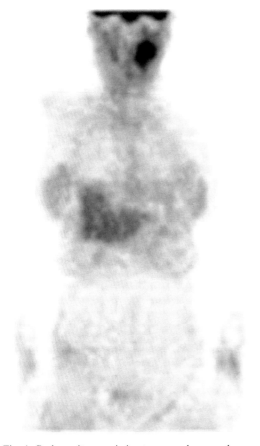

Fig. 4. Body positron emission tomography scan shows metastatic lymph nodes from an intraoral squamous cell carcinoma in the neck.

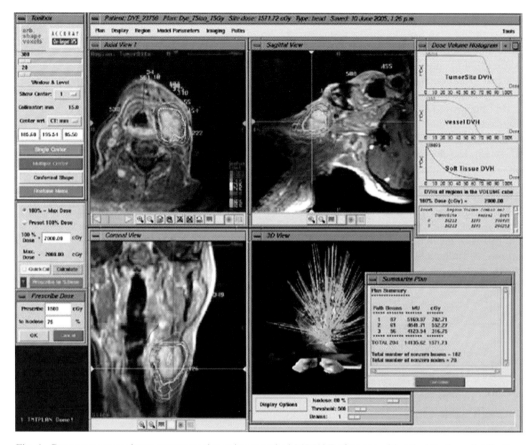

Fig. 6. Computer screen shows treatment plan using morphed MRI/CT of tumor with calculate dose distribution.

The extent of tumor repopulation kinetics during a course of radiotherapy is a determinant of radiotherapy outcome; split course radiotherapy and prolonged overall treatment time can be disadvantages in certain tumors of the head and neck region [19]. Increasing evidence indicates that this effect is caused by accelerated tumor cell repopulation.

Accelerated fractionation is a technique in which two or even three radiotherapy fractions are given per day during all or part of the treatment. This approach results in a shorter duration of radiotherapy without reducing the total dose. To allow time for repair of normal tissues, it is important to have an interval of at least 6 hours between fractions. Major cooperative trials are currently investigating dose escalation in an attempt to improve local tumor control [20,21]. These trials indicate that the decreased radiation toxicity attained by more focused delivery and the more aggressive radiation fractionation

regimens—particularly with concurrent chemotherapy—are demonstrating lessened acute radiation effects. This fact is readily recognized by the preservation of normal organ function and less involvement of normal structures and tissues proximal to the tumor [16].

Targeting tumors and avoiding proximal structures is possible because of improvements in radiation delivery by stereotactic techniques. These focused eradiation modalities include the gamma knife, CyberKnife, linear accelerator X knife, intensity moderated radiation therapy, and particle (proton ion) therapy.

The CyberKnife represents one of the most advanced radiosurgical systems available, especially for extracranial tumors (Fig. 7). Three major advantages of these newer radiosurgical systems, such as the CyberKnife, are (1) the ability to delivery a non-isocentric beam, (2) the ability to deliver pinpointed, accurate image guidance with the aid of a custom-made immobilization device

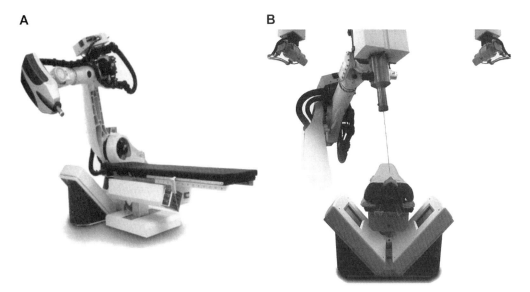

Fig. 7. (*A*) CyberKnife linear accelerator on a robotic arm. (*B*) CyberKnife with patient in dosing position.

for the head or body (Fig. 8), and (3) the capability of advanced computer software to integrate both technologies within a robotic delivery system.

Brachytherapeutic irradiation (interstitial implantation) also has been improved by the incorporation of the same three-dimensional reconstruction and localization techniques mentioned earlier. New radioisotopes, such as cesium-137 and iridium-192, have replaced the initial radium sources. These newer sources produce gamma irradiation in the kilovoltage range instead of megavolt radiation. Radiation protection devices are more predictable. The specific activity of the radiation sources can be adjusted, which enables the development of medium and

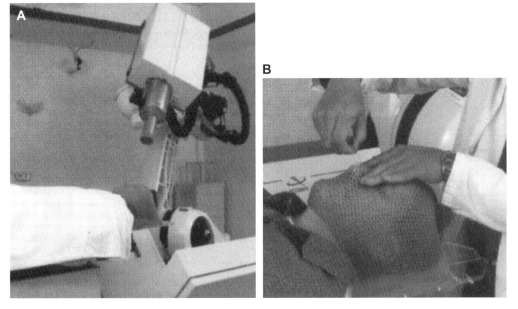

Fig. 8. (*A*) CyberKnife and patient with custom-made immobilization device. (*B*) Patient with custom-made immobilization device.

higher dose rate treatments so patients can be treated over a number of hours or minutes rather than days.

Intensity moderated radiation therapy is the most recent and advanced form of external beam radiotherapy. It has the ability to use a three-dimensional conformal delivery. Conformal radiotherapy refers to radiotherapy that has benefited from technologic developments in three-dimensional treatment planning and verification. This process allows for the high-dose regions to conform to the shape of the target volume with a minimized dose to the surrounding normal tissues and enables delivery of a higher dose per fraction (Fig. 9) [22].

In addition to improved technologies in external beam radiotherapy and brachytherapy, another tool used in conjunction with these techniques is spacers. Spacers decrease exposure of uninvolved adjacent tissues, especially the lingual aspect of the mandible, when implanted rods and pins are used [23]. Mandibular spacers are protectors that maintain the distance between the soft tissue and the mandible. Initially spacers were insertions of wet gauze—cotton "cigarette rolls"—placed between the tongue and mandible. These spacers were not steadily locked into a set position, so their effect was not dependable. It was difficult to estimate the shielded dose or dose rate absorbed by the mandible [23]. Improvements in spacer construction using acrylic resins

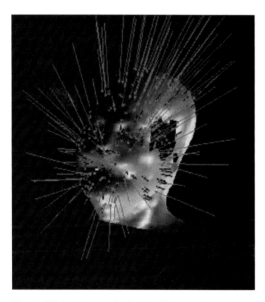

Fig. 9. Digital image of calculated beams for conforming dose of XRT.

and formal prosthesis provided a more stable and predictable placement and shield. Combined with adjunctive nutrition techniques (ie, feeding tubes), spacers can be left in place during the entire brachytherapy treatment. Studies using different spacer thicknesses demonstrated that a thickness of 7 to 10 mm (the thicker the better) can reduce the absorbed dose to the adjacent mandible by 50%. One study showed that the incidence of ORN of the lingual aspect of the mandible with spacers was 2.1% (1 out of 48) and without spacers was 40% (22 out of 55) [23].

With the combination of advancing science related to radiotherapy delivery and dose protocols, there is great hope that ORN of the mandible and other acute and long-term sequelae to normal tissues will steadily decrease and the entity of ORN will no longer be a dilemma for oral and maxillofacial surgeons.

References

[1] Rosenthal DI, Machtay M. Radiation therapy for head and neck cancer. In: Fonseca R, editor. Oral and maxillofacial surgery. Philadelphia: WB Saunders Company; 2000. p. 20–51.

[2] Marx RE, Stern D. Oral and maxillofacial pathology: a rationale for diagnosis and treatment. Carol Stream (IL): Quintessence Publishing Company, Inc; 2003. p. 375–94.

[3] Marx RE, Johnson RP. Studies in the radiobiology of osteonecrosis and their clinical significance. Oral Surg Oral Med Oral Pathol 1987;64(4):379–90.

[4] Hussey D. Principles of radiation oncology. In: Bailey BJ, editor. Head and neck surgery: otolaryngology. Philadelphia: J.B. Lippincott Company; 1993. p. 1040–9.

[5] Fletcher GH. The role of irradiation in the treatment of squamous cell carcinoma in the mouth and throat. In: Nahun AM, Bush S, Davidson TM, editors. Head and neck surgery. Boston: Mifflin Professional Publishers; 1979. p. 441.

[6] Hall EJ. Radiobiology for the radiologist. 3rd edition. Philadelphia: J.B. Lippincott; 1988.

[7] Baily BJ, Johnson JT. Head and neck surgery: otolaryngology. Philadelphia: J.B. Lippincott Company; 1997. p. 1040–8.

[8] Brown JM. Evidence for acutely hypoxic cells in mouse tumors and a possible mechanism for regeneration. Br J Radiol 1979;52:650–8.

[9] Fletcher GH. Basic principles of radiotherapy: basic clinical parameters. In: Fletcher GH, editor. Textbook of radiotherapy. Philadelphia: Lee and Febiger; 1980. p. 180–93.

[10] Ellis E. Management of the patient undergoing radiotherapy or chemotherapy. In: Peterson LJ, Ellis E, Hupp JR, et al, editors. Contemporary oral

and maxillofacial surgery. 4th edition. St. Louis: Mosby Publishing Co; 2002. p. 405–16.

[11] Marx RE. Osteoradionecrosis of the jaws [review and update]. Hyperbaric oxygen review 1984;5(2): 78–126.

[12] Tifferinton WP. Osteomyelitis and osteonecrosis of the jaws. J Oral Med 1971;26(1):7–16.

[13] Epstein JB, Wong FLW, Stevenson, et al. Osteoradionecrosis: clinical experience and a proposal for classification. J Oral Maxillofac Surg 1987;45:104–10.

[14] Marx RE, Johnson R, Kline SN. Prevention of osteoradionecrosis: a randomized prospective clinical trial of hyperbaric oxygen versus penicillin. J Am Dent Assoc 1985;111:49–54.

[15] Thornton A, Laramore G. Technical advances in radiotherapy of head and neck tumors. Hematol Oncol Clin North Am 1999;13(4):811–3.

[16] Russell NS, Bartelink H. Radiotherapy: the last 25 years. Cancer Treat Rev 1999;25(6):365–76.

[17] Nguyen LN, Ang KK. Radiotherapy for cancer of the head and neck: altered fractionation regimens. Lancet Oncol 2002;3(11):693–701.

[18] Sanders MI, Dische S, Barnett A, et al. A randomized multicenter trial of continuous hyperfractionated accelerated radiotherapy (CHART) versus conventional radiotherapy in head and neck cancer. Radiother Oncol 1997;44:123–36.

[19] Overgaard J, Helm-Hansen M, Vendello Johansen L. Comparison of conventional and split course radiotherapy as primary treatment of carcinoma of the larynx. Acta Oncol 1988;27:147–52.

[20] Ang KK. Altered fractionation trials in head and neck cancer. Semin Radiat Oncol 1998;8(4): 230–6.

[21] Horoit JC, Bontemps P, van den Bogaert W. Accelerated fractionation (AF) compared to conventional fractionation (CF) improves loco-regional control in radiotherapy of advanced head and neck cancers: results of the EORTC 22851 randomized trial. Radiother Oncol 1997;44:111–21.

[22] Ozyigit G, Chan KS. Clinical experience of head and neck cancer IMRT serial tomography. Med Dosim 2002;27(2):91–8.

[23] Masahiko M, Masamune T, Takehito S. Factors affecting mandibular complications in low dose rate brachytherapy for oral tongue carcinoma with special reference to spacer. Int J Radiat Oncol Biol Phys 1988;41(4):763–70.

ELSEVIER
SAUNDERS

Oral Maxillofacial Surg Clin N Am 19 (2007) 565–574

ORAL AND
MAXILLOFACIAL
SURGERY CLINICS
of North America

Distraction Osteogenesis: Advancements in the Last 10 Years

Joseph E. Van Sickels, DDS

*Oral & Maxillofacial Surgery, University of Kentucky College of Dentistry, 800 Rose Street,
D-508, Lexington, KY 40536-0297, USA*

The concepts of distraction osteogenesis in the maxillofacial region are similar in many respects to those used for long bones, yet differences in the shape, development, and configuration of the bones of the face make its use more challenging than traditional osteotomies. When distraction is accomplished in the maxillofacial region, several additional hard and soft tissues are also affected by the distraction process, including the teeth, gingiva, muscles, encased neural structures, temporomandibular joint, and numerous other structures in the maxilla and the mandible. Changes in the structure of the oral cavity brought about by distraction can affect breathing, speech, swallowing, and chewing, to name a few of the functional aspects of this portion of the anatomy.

The principles of distraction as refined by Ilizarov and other orthopedic surgeons continue to be refined when used by orthopedic and maxillofacial surgeons [1–4]. An almost bewildering array of appliances is available to distract the bones of the face, including intraoral and extraoral appliances, univectors and multivectors, and tooth-borne and bone-borne appliances. Each has its advantages and disadvantages. Numerous factors, including the age and nutritional state of the patient, the rate and frequency of distraction, and design of the distractor, can have tremendous impact on the quantity and quality of the bone [1–5].

Concepts

Distraction osteogenesis is an alternative technique to lengthen a bone or segment of bone by producing tensional forces at a site of surgically produced disruption. As described by Ilizarov, factors that are important for the formation of new bone are maximum preservation of extraosseous and medullary blood supply, stable fixation, a delay before distraction (latency), a distraction rate of 1 mm/d in frequent small steps (rhythm), and a period of consolidation [2]. New bone created between segments is often called the "regenerate." As seen in later sections, either during distraction or before the regenerate has consolidated, there is the capability of moving segments into a more ideal position. Ilizarov evaluated the influence of the rate and frequency of distraction on osteogenesis during limb elongation in a canine model [1]. Using distraction rates of 0.5, 1, or 2 mm/d and different distraction frequencies with both osteotomies and closed techniques, he found that a distraction rate of 1 mm/d led to the best results for bone, fascia, skeletal muscles, smooth muscle, blood vessels, nerves, and skin. When he used a rate of 0.5 mm/d, it often led to premature consolidation of the lengthening bone, whereas a distraction rate of 2 mm/d led to undesirable changes within the elongated tissues. He observed that the greater the distraction frequency, the better the outcome. He concluded that the best results were obtained with preservation of periosseous tissues, bone marrow, and blood supply at the time of osteotomy, stability of the distractor (external), and a rate of 1 mm/d with a rhythm of four turns per day. His findings were confirmed in a review paper by Aronson [3].

In contrast, Troulis and colleagues [6] used a porcine model to distract the mandible varying both latency and the rate of distraction. They found that the most successful model used a rate of 1 mm/d without a latency period. Hollier and colleagues [7] used no latency periods and faster

E-mail address: vansick@email.uky.edu

distraction rates in a pediatric population. These last two papers may represent differences seen when working in the maxillofacial region and with a pediatric population.

Histology

From a histologic evaluation, when distraction is completed, new bone forms in parallel columns that extend in both directions from the osteotomy [1]. The distraction process can be divided into three phases [8]. During the latency period (first phase), histologic and molecular events are similar to those seen during fracture healing, with the osteotomy site surrounded by a hyaline cartilage external callus. In the distraction phase (second phase), chondrocytes are stretched along the tension vector and become fibroblast-like in shape. As distraction is advanced (third phase), the cartilaginous callus is progressively replaced by a bone callus first by endochrondral ossification; later new bone is directly formed by intramembranous ossification. During distraction, several molecules of the bone morphogenic protein super family have been noted [9]. Several studies have noted increased blood flow and vessel formation within the zone of distraction [10]. Pacicca and colleagues [10] showed two different angiogenic factors localized at the leading edge of the distraction gap where new bone was forming. They also found these factors to be maximal during active distraction.

In a study of animal distraction of the mandible, Glowacki and colleagues [11] noted that bone fill was significantly correlated with clinical stability and exuberant periosteal osteogenesis was present, which prompted them to suggest that the periosteum was a major source of new bone formation. Mackool and colleagues [12] analyzed the mandibles of five patients who underwent unilateral or bilateral distraction with CT scans. They found that the segmental volumes of the distracted mandibles were of similar or greater volume when compared with the preoperative mandibular segments, and the distribution of regenerate bone was similar to the physiologic preoperative bone. In a similar study, they found that there was an increase in the volume of the attached muscles [13].

Animal models and clinical studies have shown that it is possible to manipulate immature bone before it completely consolidates [14,15]. This finding is particularly helpful in the maxillofacial complex, in which occlusal discrepancies are difficult to manage once the bone has healed

completely. Clinically this is called "molding the regenerate." (See the section on distraction in the maxillofacial region.)

Thurmuller and colleagues [16] found that high rates of distraction had adverse effects on the temporomandibular joints of minipigs. Others have found that the temporomandibular joint responds well to normal distraction rate and rhythm [17]. One case of condylar resorption after mandibular advancement by distraction osteogenesis was reported, however [18]. Although controversial, it is likely that distraction—particularly with frequent rhythm—is more physiologically "kind" to joints than dramatic translocations of segments seen with traditional osteotomies, especially in patients who have unstable joints.

Variables

Variables are numerous and include rate and rhythm, age of the patient, systemic factors, type of distractor, and bone being distracted.

Rate and rhythm

In practice, most surgeons use a 3- to 5-day latency period followed by a rate of 1 mm/d with a twice-a-day rhythm in the mandible. A shorter latency is used in the maxilla.

Age of the patient

Aronson and colleagues [4] looked at distraction of the tibia in two different groups of rats to study the effects of age using videomicroscopy to quantitate radiodensity, histology, and relative areas of cellular proliferation. In both groups they saw an age-related decrease in the percent of mineralized bone density. In a pediatric population, Hollier and colleagues [7] were able to eliminate the latency period and successfully distracted the mandibles of 22 patients at a rate of 2 mm/d. Most surgeons use a shorter latency in pediatric patients and a more rapid rate of expansion. One of the complications of a long latency or a slow distraction rate in a pediatric population is premature consolidation.

Systemic factors

Numerous known systemic factors can affect distraction. One of the more frequently studied ones is chronic ethanol use [5,19–22]. Just as chronic alcohol abuse is associated with increases in incidence of fracture and complication with fracture healing, it decreases bone regeneration seen with distraction osteogenesis [5,20–22]. Interesting work has shown that the inhibition demonstrated by chronic ethanol exposure in a rat model is attenuated by the simultaneous administration of antagonist to the cytokines interleukin-1β and tumor necrosis factor-α [5,22]. In a small series of cases of maxillary distraction with internal distractors, Van Sickels and colleagues [23] reported one case of a nonunion after maxillary distraction in which the patient was HIV positive, hepatitis C positive, had previous cleft lip and palate surgery, and had a history of smoking and alcohol use. Although the patient did achieve a union after a Le Fort I osteotomy with a bone graft, it is unknown which of these factors or combination of them contributed to his nonunion. Although each of the factors had a negative effect on bone healing, none of them represented an absolute contraindication to distraction osteogenesis. The ideal management of patients with history of smoking and alcohol use involves eliminating or markedly reducing their use before surgery.

Type of distractor

The number of different types of distractors that are available is beyond the scope of this article; however, several studies have examined the biomechanics of different types of distractors. Fundamentally, external distractors are less stable than internal ones [24]. Haug and colleagues [24] studied external and internal distractors and found under biomechanical testing that external distractors failed with permanent deformation of the pins rather than fracture of the model, as seen in the ones with internal distractors. The situation becomes more complex when soft tissue considerations are made. In a separate study, Demann and Haug [25] found that the position in which the distractor is placed to simulate soft tissues affects the distraction vector. This finding is similar to clinical evaluations for mandibular advancement of the mandible [26,27]. Van Strijen and colleagues [26] evaluated 50 cases of mandibular advancement by distraction osteogenesis. They found the most stable results in low-angle cases and relapse in high-angle cases. Their findings were probably caused by deep bite seen with low-angle cases and the positive effect of the suprahyoid musculature on the results as opposed to the high-angle cases. (See case three later in article.)

Advantages to internal distractors are that they are hidden in the oral cavity and are less obvious. They are more difficulties for patients regarding oral hygiene and oral discomfort. Once the distractor is placed, it is more difficult to manage the primary vector of distraction when internal distractors are used versus external distractions (see later discussion) [23].

Vector

Vector is the direction that the segment is moved. Extrinsic and intrinsic vectors must be considered when planning a case [28]. In the case of a single vector ramus distractor, the primary vector is the direction that the tram is pointed. If the patient is mandibular deficient (class II) on one side or if the mandibular midline and the chin are off to the same side, this determines if the distractor should be placed in a strictly vertical direction or with an anterior component to the vector. (See case two later in article.) Intrinsic vectors (the masseter and medial pterygoid muscles) are more resistant to vertical movement of the segment than the suprahyoid musculature is to anterior movement of the mandible.

In contrast to vertical distraction of the ramus, with mandibular advancement the suprahyoid musculature exerts a vertical pull as the distal segment as the mandible is advanced. To counteract these intrinsic vectors, the distractors should be directed in a slightly upward direction toward the maxillary dentition. (See case four later in article.) Even with overcorrection of the primary vector, there is a tendency for an anterior open bite to occur in cases of mandibular advancement. Secondary extrinsic elastic vectors can used be during the distraction phase and early in the consolidation phase to settle the occlusion.

Distraction in the maxillofacial region

Numerous articles have been written on the use of distraction for routine and complex cases that involve segments or total arches moved to achieve functional improvement for patients [23,29–33]. Monofocal, bifocal, and even trifocal distraction has been used to lengthen the mandible or maxilla or close continuity defects of the jaws [23,33]. The primary type of distraction used in the maxillofacial region is monofocal distraction, in which the mandible or maxilla is lengthened. Because of difficulty achieving the precise occlusal results, as seen with orthognathic surgery, most surgeons try to manipulate immature bone before it has a chance to completely consolidate. This is frequently referred to as "molding the regenerate" [14,15].

Shetye and colleagues [33] evaluated 12 consecutive patients who underwent mandibular ramal distraction with a range of 5 years. They found mild relapse during the first year after distraction and long-term stability of the results. McCarthy and colleagues [15] used multivector distractors to change the primary vector and elastics to add secondary extrinsic vectors to mold the regenerate and achieve a more favorable occlusal result. It is possible to change the primary vector during the activation and consolidation periods. Although both periods are used, it is preferred to manipulate the regenerate during the activation period to minimize occlusal discrepancies. (See case three later in article.)

A discussion of the number of different types of procedures that can be accomplished with distraction and indications for all of them is beyond the scope of this article. The focus of the remaining portion of this article is on selected maxillary and mandibular advancements and segmental procedures.

Transport distraction is used in bifocal and trifocal distractions to close continuity defects. With transport distraction, a segment of vascularized bone is moved until it "docks" with the other side. A variation of this theme has been used in implant dentistry to create more bone and soft tissue [29]. (See case five later in article.) As with most of distraction, vector control can be difficult and result in less-than-desirable position for the segment. Its main indication is for height defects in the mandible but it is used especially in the "aesthetic zone" of the maxilla.

Numerous articles have been published on advancement of the mandible in children with airway difficulties or in whom tracheotomies already were used [30,31]. (See case one later in article.) Steinbacher and colleagues [30] reviewed their results after advancement of the mandible with five children aged 2 to 14 years who depended on tracheostomy. Their protocol consisted of a latency of 48 hours and a rate of 1 mm/d. They used semi-buried unidirectional devices, and their average duration of fixation was 40 to 60 days. Their average advancement was 23 mm. Four of the five patients were decannulated. The most successful results after distraction for children with obstruction of the airways have occurred in patients with Pierre Robin sequence in whom airway obstruction is supraglottic and in whom there are no additional neurologic symptoms. Schaefer and colleagues [31] felt that there were multiple options for infants with Pierre Robin sequence, including positioning, tongue lip adhesion, and distraction. They felt that if the airway obstruction was at the base of the tongue, a tongue lip adhesion should be performed first; if the procedure is unsuccessful, then distraction of the mandible should be used to avoid a tracheostomy for these patients.

Cases

Case 1: Pediatric mandibular advancement for airway issue

A 2-month-old patient who had Pierre Robin sequence and failure to thrive was assessed by pediatric, otolaryngology, and oral and maxillofacial surgery services. He was severely retrognathic and had sternal retraction with attempts to feed. A feeding tube was placed, and instructions were given to the mother as to how to manage the infant's airway. After these maneuvers, the child gained weight; at 4 months he weighed 10 pounds (Fig. 1). He was scheduled for surgery in which he underwent an extraoral inverted "L" osteotomy of his mandible and placement of external distractors (Figs. 2 and 3). A 24-hour latency period was used and he was advanced at 1.5 mm/d. His mandible was advanced 14 mm, and the distractor was stabilized for a consolidation period of 1 month. After removal of his distractors he was able to feed in a normal fashion.

Case 2: Combined ramus distraction and orthognathic surgery

A 14-year-old girl with craniofacial microsomia was referred for evaluation of her

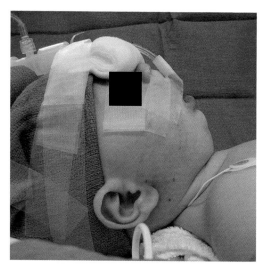

Fig. 1. Preoperative view of 4-month-old patient with Pierre Robin sequence and difficulty breathing.

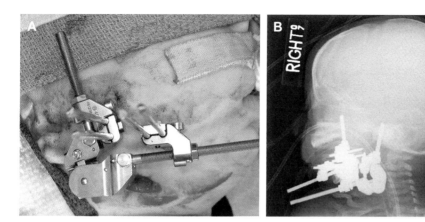

Fig. 2. (A) Intraoperative view with external distractor in place after mandibular osteotomy. (B) Radiograph obtained in the operating room with distractors in place.

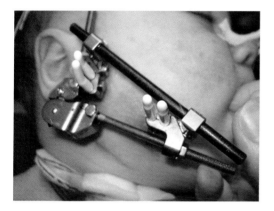

Fig. 3. After 14 mm of distraction, distractor stabilized.

dentofacial discrepancies. She had a 6-mm discrepancy between the right and left mandibular ridge heights with a significant cant in the maxilla and the maxillary midline deviated to the right (Figs. 4 and 5). The first stage of her surgery was to distract the ramus on the right side with a single vector distractor that was directed inferiorly and anteriorly. The latency was 3 days, and the distraction was 1 mm/d divided into a twice-a-day rhythm. Total distraction took 8 days, leveling the mandibular occlusal plane and shifting the mandibular midline further to the left to create more of a posterior open bite on the right (Fig. 6). After a consolidation period of 2 months, she underwent a Le Fort I osteotomy, which

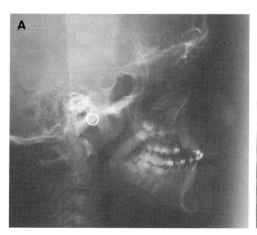

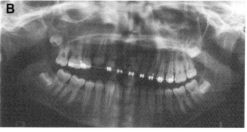

Fig. 4. (A) Lateral cephalogram of patient with craniofacial microsomia. (B) Panoramic radiograph illustrates the deficient right side.

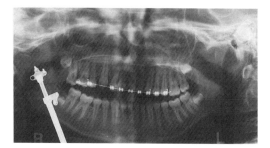

Fig. 5. Panoramic radiograph with single vector distractor in place.

leveled her maxillary occlusal plane and shifted the maxillary midline to the left.

Case 3: Maxillary advancement for cleft palate

A 15-year-old boy with partial anadontia, cleft lip and palate repair, and maxillary hypoplasia was referred for surgical correction. A lateral cephalogram reveled that he was horizontal and vertical maxillary hypoplastic (Fig. 7). He was marginally velopharyngeal competent and needed 7-mm advancement to accomplish ideal occlusal results. He had a consultation regarding deterioration of his velopharyngeal competence. A 1-mm fine-cut axial CT scan of his maxilla was obtained to generate a stereolithographic model. Internal distractors were contoured to the model to develop an anterior and inferior vector of distraction (Fig. 8). Using this vector, along with setting the trams to be at the level of the maxillary occlusal plane, minimized the oral discomfort for the patient. A 3-day latency period was used followed by a distraction rate of 1 mm/d with a twice-a-day rhythm. A total distraction time of 10 days was followed by a 2-month period of consolidation. On clinical examination, his speech

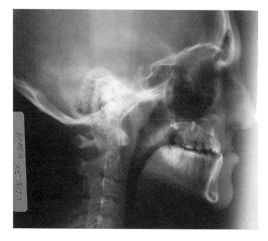

Fig. 7. Lateral cephalogram of patient with cleft lip and palate and maxillary hypoplasia.

improved and velopharyngeal function remained the same as before surgery.

Case 4: Mandibular advancement for large or complicated cases

A 17-year-old boy was referred after an unsuccessful attempt to advance the mandible by a sagittal split osteotomy (Fig. 9A, B). His overjet was 9 mm and he had a 50% overbite (Fig. 9C). The previous surgeon noted that his ramus on both sides was thin. A CT scan confirmed his finding. Three months after his first surgery he underwent distraction of his mandible with internal distractors, which were contoured on a stereolithographic model in which the primary extrinsic vector was directed superiorly toward the maxillary occlusal plane (Fig. 10A). After 10 days of distraction he still had a slight open bite tendency (Fig. 10B). Vertical elastics were placed

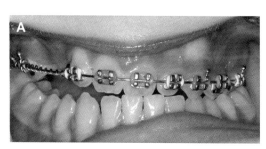
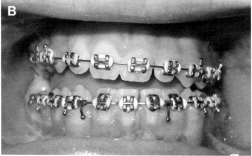

Fig. 6. (A) Preoperative occlusion. (B) Occlusion after distraction of the right side.

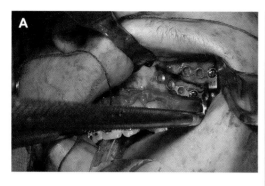
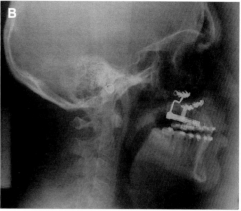

Fig. 8. (*A*) Intraoperative photographic of placement of internal distractor on left. (*B*) Lateral cephalogram of maxilla with distractors near the end of distraction.

(secondary extrinsic vectors) during the early period of consolidation, and his occlusion was satisfactory.

Case 5: Alveolar distraction

A 22-year-old woman was referred for evaluation of deficient alveolar ridges after a motor vehicle collision in which she suffered multiple facial fractures with loss of maxillary and mandibular teeth and bone (Fig. 11). The maxillary defect was more pronounced on the right side of the maxilla than the left. A transport segment was created, and an alveolar distractor was placed to the right of the midline of the segment. This procedure allowed differential movement of the right side over the left (Fig. 12). A 5-day latency was used with a 1.15-mm rate achieved by

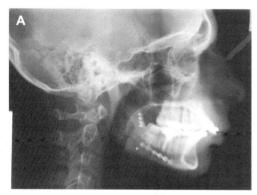
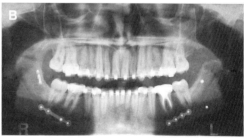
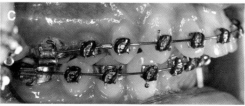

Fig. 9. (*A*) Preoperative lateral cephalogram of patient after unsuccessful mandibular advancement. (*B*) Panoramic radiograph shows stabilization with initial surgery. (*C*) Preoperative occlusion.

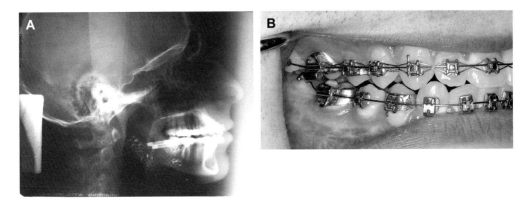

Fig. 10. (*A*) Six weeks after distraction of mandible (10 mm). (*B*) Occlusion during orthodontics after removal of distractors.

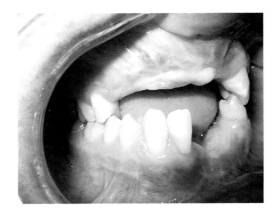

Fig. 11. Maxillary defect after motor vehicle accident with loss of height and projection.

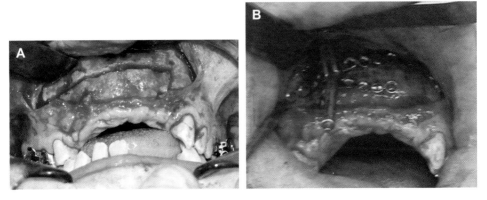

Fig. 12. (*A*) Transport disc created. (*B*) Distractor in place.

a three-times-a-day rhythm of 0.35 mm. Advancement of 12 mm was accomplished. After a 2-month consolidation period, osseointegrated implants were placed. Because of an infection in the mandible at the time of the maxillary procedure, mandibular distraction was then undertaken (Fig. 13).

Summary

Distraction is still evolving in the management of patients with orthopedic and craniomaxillofacial deformities. The relationship among latency, gap size, rate, rhythm, and duration of fixation is not totally understood for all of the individual patients and variations in their needs seen in a clinical practice. Numerous factors can influence the quality and quantity of bone seen with distraction, including the age and nutritional status of the patient and the type of distractor that is used. Although the ideal rate of distraction seems to be 1 mm/d in a healthy adult, a much more rapid rate of 1.5 to 2 mm in a pediatric population seems to give acceptable results. Likewise, a latency period of 3 to 7 days is customary in adults but is unnecessary in the pediatric population. In contrast, in older patients or patients for whom alcohol may be a problem, longer latency periods, slower distraction rates, and longer consolidation periods may be necessary. The mandible in adults is more like the long bones of the extremities. In contrast, the maxilla has more medullary bone and a richer blood supply, and it probably needs less of a latency period and can be moved at a faster rate than the

mandible. The position in which the distractor is placed and the overlying soft tissue have considerable influence on the vector of distraction, which can be used as an advantage when bone and soft tissue defects are irregular. Because of the precise nature of the occlusion, manipulation of the regenerate either during the active phase of distraction or early in consolidation frequently is necessary.

References

[1] Ilizarov GA. The tension-stress effect on the genesis and growth of tissues. Part II. The influence of the rate and frequency of distraction. Clin Orthop Relat Res 1989;239:263–85.

[2] Ilizarov GA. Clinical application of the tension-stress effect for limb lengthening. Clin Orthop Relat Res 1990;250:8–26.

[3] Aronson J. Experimental and clinical experience with distraction osteogenesis. Cleft Palate Craniofac J 1994;31:473–81.

[4] Aronson J, Gao GG, Shen XC, et al. The effect of aging on distraction osteogenesis in the rat. J Orthop Res 2001;19:421–7.

[5] Wahl EC, Perrien DS, Aronson J, et al. Ethanol-induced inhibition of bone formation in a rat model of distraction osteogenesis: a role for the tumor necrosis factor signaling axis. Alcohol Clin Exp Res 2005;29:1466–72.

[6] Troulis MJ, Glowacki J, Perrott DH, et al. Effects of latency and rate on bone formation in a porcine mandibular distraction model. J Oral Maxillofac Surg 2000;58:507–13.

[7] Hollier LH Jr, Higuera S, Stal S, et al. Distraction rate and latency: factors in the outcome of pediatric mandibular distraction. Plast Reconstr Surg 2006; 117:2333–6.

[8] Sato M, Yasui N, Nakase T, et al. Expression of bone matrix proteins mRNA during distraction osteogenesis. J Bone Miner Res 1998;13:1221–31.

[9] Sato M, Ochi T, Nakase T, et al. Mechanical tension-stress induces expression of bone morphogenic protein (BMP)-2 and BMP-4, but not BMP-6, BMP-7, and GDF5 mRNA, during distraction osteogenesis. J Bone Miner Res 1999;14:1084–95.

[10] Pacicca DM, Patel N, Lee C, et al. Expression of angiogenic factors during distraction osteogenesis. Bone 2003;33:889–98.

[11] Glowacki J, Shusterman EM, Troulis M, et al. Distraction osteogenesis of the porcine mandible: histomorphometric evaluation of bone. Plast Reconstr Surg 2004;113:566–73.

[12] Mackool RJ, Grayson BH, McCarthy JG. Volumetric assessment of the distracted human mandible. J Craniofac Surg 2004;15:745–50.

[13] Mackool RJ, Hooper RA, Grayson BH, et al. Volumetric change of the medial pterygoid following

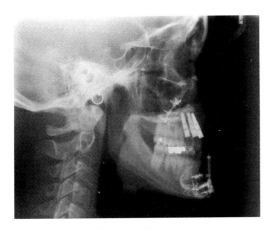

Fig. 13. Twelve millimeters of distraction and placement of implants in the maxilla, distraction begun in the mandible.

distraction osteogenesis of the mandible: an example of the associated soft tissue changes. Plast Reconstr Surg 2003;111:1804–7.

[14] Luchs JS, Steinicki EJ, Rowe N, et al. Molding of the regenerate in mandibular distraction. Part I. Laboratory study. J Craniofac Surg 2002;13:205–11.

[15] McCarthy JG, Hopper RA, Hollier LH Jr, et al. Molding of the regenerate in mandibular distraction: clinical experience. Plast Reconstr Surg 2003;112:1239–46.

[16] Thurmuller P, Troulis MJ, Rosenberg A, et al. Microscopic changes in the condyle and disc in response to distraction osteogenesis of the minipig mandible. J Oral Maxillofac Surg 2006;64:249–58.

[17] Steinichi EJ, Stucki-McCormick SU, Rowe N, et al. Remodeling of the temporomandibular joint following mandibular distraction osteogenesis in the transverse dimension. Plast Reconstr Surg 2001;107:647–58.

[18] van Strijen PJ, Breuning KH, Becking AG, et al. Condylar resorption following distraction osteogenesis: a case report. J Oral Maxillofac Surg 2001;59:1104–7.

[19] Wahl EC, Liu L, Perrien DS, et al. A novel mouse model for the study of the inhibitory effects of chronic ethanol on direct bone formation. Alcohol 2006;39:159–67.

[20] Chakkalakal DA, Novak JR, Fritz ED, et al. Inhibition of bone repair in a rat model for chronic and excessive alcohol consumption. Alcohol 2005;36:210–4.

[21] Brown EC, Perrien DS, Fletcher TW, et al. Skeletal toxicity associated with chronic ethanol exposure in a rat model using total enteral nutrition. J Pharmacol Exp Ther 2002;301:1132–8.

[22] Perrien DS, Brown EC, Fletcher TW, et al. Interleukin-1 and tumor necrosis factor antagonist attenuate ethanol induced inhibition of bone formation in a rat model of distraction osteogenesis. J Pharmacol Exp Ther 2002;303:904–8.

[23] Van Sickels JE, Madsen MJ, Cunningham LL Jr, et al. The use of internal maxillary distraction for maxillary hypoplasia: a preliminary report. J Oral Maxillofac Surg 2006;64:1715–20.

[24] Haug RH, Nuveen EJ, Barber JE, et al. An in vitro evaluation of distractors used for osteogenesis. Oral Surg Oral Med Oral Pathol Oral Radiol Endod 1998;86:648–59.

[25] Demann ET, Haug RH. Do position and soft tissue affect distraction vector? An in vitro investigation. J Oral Maxillofac Surg 2002;60:149–66.

[26] van Strijen PJ, Breuning KH, Becking AG, et al. Stability after distraction osteogenesis to lengthen the mandible: results in 50 cases. J Oral Maxillofac Surg 2004;62:304–7.

[27] Hendrickx K, Mommaerts M, Jacobs W, et al. Proximal segment position after distraction with the MD-DOS device. J Craniomaxillofac Surg 1999;27:383–6.

[28] Van Sickels JE. Distraction osteogenesis versus orthognathic surgery. Am J Orthod Dentofacial Orthop 2000;118:482–4.

[29] Jensen OT, Cockrell R, Kuhike L, et al. Anterior maxillary alveolar distraction osteogenesis: a prospective 5 year clinical study. Int J Oral Maxillofac Implants 2002;17:52–68.

[30] Steinbacher DM, Kaban LB, Troulis MJ. Mandibular advancement by distraction osteogenesis for tracheostomy dependent children with severe micrognathia. J Oral Maxillofac Surg 2005;63:1072–9.

[31] Schaefer RB, Stadler JA 3rd, Gosain AK. To distract or not to distract: an algorithm for airway management in isolated Pierre Robin sequence. Plast Reconstr Surg 2004;113:1113–25.

[32] Eski M, Turegun M, Deveci M, et al. Vertical distraction osteogenesis of fibular bone flap in reconstructed mandible. Ann Plast Surg 2006;57:631–6.

[33] Shetye PR, Grayson BH, Mackool RJ, et al. Long term stability and growth following unilateral mandibular distraction in growing children with craniofacial microsomia. Plast Reconstr Surg 2006;118:985–95.

ELSEVIER
SAUNDERS

Oral Maxillofacial Surg Clin N Am 19 (2007) 575–589

**ORAL AND
MAXILLOFACIAL
SURGERY CLINICS**
of North America

Bone Morphogenetic Proteins and the Induction of Bone Formation: From Laboratory to Patients

Ugo Ripamonti, MD, PhD[a,b,*],
Manolis Heliotis, MBChB, BDS, MSc, FDSRCS, FRCS[c],
Carlo Ferretti, DDS, MDent, FCD(SA)MFOS[d]

[a]*Bone Research Unit, Medical Research Council/University of the Witwatersrand,
Medical School, 2193 Parktown, Johannesburg, South Africa*
[b]*School of Clinical Medicine, Faculty of Health Sciences, University of the Witwatersrand,
Medical School, 2193 Parktown, Johannesburg, South Africa*
[c]*North West London Regional Maxillofacial Unit, Northwick Park Hospital, London, UK*
[d]*Division of Maxillofacial and Oral Surgery, Chris Hani Baragwanath Hospital,
University of the Witwatersrand, Johannesburg, South Africa*

The osteogenic soluble molecular signals of the transforming growth factor-β (TGF-β) superfamily—the bone morphogenetic/osteogenic proteins (BMPs/OPs)—induce endochondral bone formation as a recapitulation of embryonic development and uniquely in primates the TGF-β isoforms per se [1–3]. Together with the soluble molecular signals, regenerative medicine in craniomandibulofacial surgery starts by erecting scaffolds of biomimetic biomaterial matrices that mimic the supramolecular assembly of the extracellular matrix of bone [3,4]. Naturally derived BMPs/OPs and gamma-irradiated human recombinant osteogenic protein-1 (hOP-1) delivered by allogeneic and xenogeneic insoluble collagenous bone matrices initiate the induction of bone formation in heterotopic extraskeletal and orthotopic skeletal sites of the nonhuman primate *Papio ursinus*. This process culminates in complete calvarial regeneration by day 90 and maintains the regenerated constructs by day 365 [3–6]. The induction of

bone by hOP-1 in *Papio ursinus* develops as a mosaic structure with distinct spatial and temporal patterns of gene expression of members of the TGF-β superfamily that singly, synergistically, and synchronously initiate and maintain tissue induction and morphogenesis [3,7].

Highly purified, naturally derived BMPs/OPs and hOP-1 delivered by collagenous bone matrices and porous hydroxyapatite, respectively, induce bone formation in mandibular defects of human patients. Clinical trials have used doses that are many times higher than the doses suggested by the results in animal models, including nonhuman primates. Supraphysiologic doses of single recombinant gene proteins suggest a flaw in the single morphogen approach to human osteoinduction. The induction of bone by available single recombinant human BMPs/OPs (ie, BMP-2 and OP-1) is too costly because of the high doses required to induce an often comparatively mediocre regenerated osseous construct in clinical contexts. In humans, the induction of bone is on a different scale compared with animal models, including nonhuman primate species.

The induction of bone formation can be enhanced significantly by the synergistic induction of bone formation, however, in which relatively low doses of TGF-β isoforms synergize with hOP-1 to initiate rapid and substantial bone formation in heterotopic and orthotopic sites of the nonhuman

Supported by the South African Medical Research Council, the University of the Witwatersrand, Johannesburg and the National Research Foundation.

* Corresponding author. Bone Research Unit, Medical Research Council/University of the Witwatersrand, Medical School, 2193 Parktown, Johannesburg, South Africa.

E-mail address: ugo.ripamonti@wits.ac.za
(U. Ripamonti).

primate *Papio ursinus* [3–5]. The time has now arrived to move into the clinical arena to translate research results in clinical contexts of regenerative medicine and strategize that the synergistic induction of bone formation is the novel therapeutic strategy for axial and craniomandibulofacial reconstruction, particularly in elderly persons, in whom repair phenomena are often limited because of recipient bed deficiencies, such as poor vascularity, chronic irradiation, fibrosis, infection, and usually lack of freshly available responding cells.

This article reviews the induction of bone by the osteogenic proteins of the TGF-β superfamily in nonhuman and human primates and proposes that the translation in clinical contexts of the phenomenon of bone formation by autoinduction is predictably achievable by the binary application of relatively low doses of TGF-β proteins with a recombinant human osteogenic protein. In primates, the induction of bone formation develops as a mosaic structure in which the osteogenic proteins of the TGF-β superfamily singly, synergistically, and synchronously initiate and maintain tissue induction and morphogenesis [3–5]. TGF-β proteins induce bone formation in primates only. The synergistic induction of bone formation is a cost-effective clinical strategy because published data in nonhuman primates have shown that doses of recombinant hOP-1 can be reduced at least fivefold and still increase bone formation compared with higher doses of single applications of hOP-1 [8–10].

Bone: formation by autoinduction

Bone formation by induction refers to a developmental cascade of molecular and cellular events in which heterotopic intramuscular or subcutaneous implantation of demineralized bone matrix results in the endochondral induction of bone formation within the implanted matrix [1–3]. Since the classic studies of Levander, Moss, Trueta, and Urist during last century [11], significant research outputs have cast the principles for regenerative medicine and tissue engineering of bone and have identified novel molecular therapeutics endowed with the striking prerogative to initiate heterotopic induction of bone formation (Fig. 1) [3–5]. Which molecular signals are endowed with the striking prerogative of initiating de novo bone formation by induction in heterotopic extraskeletal sites? Which molecular signals are capable of interacting with responding mesenchymal stem cells to induce chondroblastic and osteoblastic phenotypes and induce de novo endochondral bone later to be mineralized facing foci of hematopoietic bone marrow within the newly formed heterotopic ossicles?

The fundamental work of Huggins, Levander, Moss, Trueta, Urist, and Reddi [11] has dramatically indicated that the extracellular matrices of bone and dentine contain morphogenetic signals endowed with the striking prerogative of initiating bone formation by induction in heterotopic extraskeletal sites of animal models, including primates [1–11]. The presence of putative osteogenic proteins was a challenge for more than a century since the published work of Senn and later Sacerdotti and Frattin on the induction of bone formation in the kidney upon ligature of the renal artery [11]. Building on previously published experimental work by Levander, Lacroix, Levander and Willestaedt, Bridges and Pritchard, and Moss, Urist, borrowing the term "induction" from Spemann [12] and Levander [13], produced evidence that intramuscular implantation of demineralized bone matrix in heterotopic intramuscular sites results in bone formation by autoinduction [14].

Mineralized matrices of bone and dentin contain signaling molecules ("morphogens"), as defined by Turing [15], that are capable of imparting differentiating pathways to responding cells after interaction with specific cell surface receptors, initiating the ripple-like cascade of pattern formation and the generation of bone with hematopoietic bone marrow [1–3,16]. How to access and isolate the morphogens responsible for the induction of bone? The biochemical problem of the putative osteogenic proteins tightly bound to the extracellular matrix of bone was unlocked by the solubilization of bone-inductive protein fractions from the bone matrix [17]. This critical experiment showed that the intact demineralized bone matrix could be dissociatively extracted with chaotropic agents yielding solubilized proteins and a residual inactive insoluble collagenous bone matrix [17]. The realization that intact demineralized bone matrix could be dissociatively extracted and inactivated and that the osteogenic activity restored by reconstituting the inactive residue with solubilized protein fractions [17] made possible the development and application of increasingly refined purification schemes that mainly involved liquid chromatography on the solubilized protein fractions [18–21].

Importantly for tissue engineering strategies in clinical contexts, neither the solubilized proteins nor the insoluble collagenous matrix residue were active [17,22]; however, a combination of the two components restored the osteogenic activity in

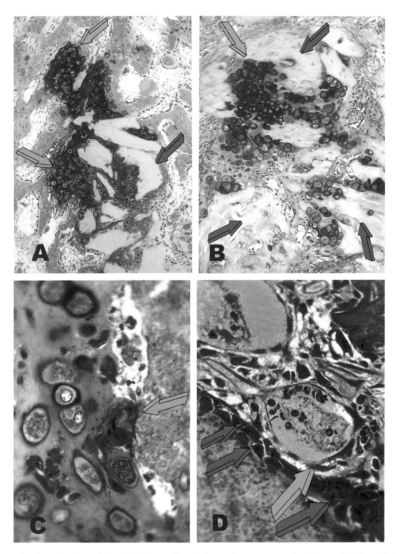

Fig. 1. Soluble molecular signals and the induction of bone formation as a recapitulation of embryonic development in the rat heterotopic bioassay after subcutaneous implantation of 5 to 20 μg of highly purified baboon bone-derived BMPs/OPs (*A, B*) and 0.1 to 0.5 μg of gel-eluted osteogenic proteins purified to apparent homogeneity (*C, D*) (*A*) Cartilage anlages (*blue arrows*) surrounded by matrix particles (*red arrow*) and newly formed trabeculae of bone. (*B*) Scattered islands of newly formed cartilage (*blue arrow*) with matrix particles (*red arrows*) and vascular invasion precipitating chondrolysis or death of the cartilage. (*C*) Induction of chondrogenesis attached to the matrix carrier (*blue arrow*). (*D*) Induction of osteoblastic cell differentiation attached to the matrix (*red arrows*) with capillary invasion and angiogenesis. Intimate relationships between differentiating osteoblastic cells and the invading capillary with migrating endothelial cells from the vascular compartment (*blue arrow*) to the bone forming osteoblastic microenvironment as precursor osteogenic cells. Original magnification: (*A, B*) ×125; (*C*) ×460; (*D*) ×270.

the extraskeletal heterotopic bioassay (Fig. 1) [1,3,17,22,23]. This operational reconstitution of the soluble signal with an insoluble substratum was a key experiment that provided a bioassay for bona fide initiators of endochondral bone differentiation [1,3]. It was noteworthy that the induction of bone formation in the rodent heterotopic assay was also possible after the reconstitution of rat insoluble collagenous bone matrix with solubilized osteogenic proteins of different mammalian species (Fig. 1C, D) [22]. These classic experiments implied that there are homologies between bone-inductive proteins from human, baboon, monkey, bovine, and rat extracellular matrices [22]. The operational reconstitution of the soluble signal with an insoluble substratum was a key experiment that provided a bioassay for bona fide initiators of endochondral bone differentiation [1,3,23] and set a race for the purification of an entirely new family of protein initiators collectively called BMPs/OPs, which belong to the TGF-β superfamily [1–3,24]. The classic experiments of Sampath and Reddi [17,22] also highlighted the critical role of recombining or reconstituting the osteogenic soluble molecular signal with an insoluble signal or substratum to trigger the bone induction cascade [1,3,17,22,23].

When writing about osteoinduction, it is important to define properly the terminology related to bone formation by autoinduction [1,4,17,22,23]. The acid test of the induction of bone formation is the de novo generation of bone in heterotopic extraskeletal sites of animal models after extraskeletal implantation of the osteogenic soluble molecular signals of the TGF-β superfamily [1,3,23]. A protein labeled as osteoinductive must be endowed with the striking capacity of initiating endochondral bone formation in heterotopic extraskeletal sites (Fig. 1) [1,3,23]. The heterotopic implantation sites avoid the ambiguities of the orthotopic site in which bone formation by conduction may occur from the viable bone interfaces, particularly when using osteophilic porous substrata as bone repair materials [3,14].

Whether the biologic activity of partially purified BMPs/OPs, as shown in long-term experiments in the adult nonhuman primate *Papio ursinus* (Fig. 2), is the result of the sum of a plurality of BMP/OP activities or a truly synergistic interaction amongst different BMPs/OPs deserves appropriate investigation [3,6,10]. In the identical orthotopic model, however, the long-term efficacy of single applications of gamma-irradiated hOP-1 delivered by a bovine collagenous matrix in regenerating large calvarial defects of membranous bone of the adult primate was demonstrated (Fig. 3) [6,25]. Morphologic analyses on undecalcified sections showed that doses of hOP-1, recombined with gamma-irradiated bovine collagenous bone matrix, induced the complete regeneration of nonhealing calvarial defects, which maintained the architecture of the newly formed bone up to 1 year after implantation (Fig. 3) [3,6,25].

Synergistic induction of bone formation

Importantly and conclusively, in the bona fide bioassay for bone induction in rodents, the TGF-β isoforms do not initiate the induction of bone formation [26]. In marked contrast to the results obtained in rodents, however, the mammalian TGF-β isoforms and even the amphibian TGF-β$_5$ isoform [4] do induce endochondral bone formation when implanted in heterotopic extraskeletal sites of the nonhuman primate *Papio ursinus* (Fig. 4A) [8–11].

The pleiotropy of the signaling molecules of the TGF-β superfamily is highlighted by the apparent redundancy of molecular signals initiating endochondral bone induction but in the primate only [8–11]. The TGF-β isoforms are powerful inducers of endochondral bone when implanted in the *rectus abdominis* muscle of the nonhuman primate *Papio ursinus* at doses of 5, 25, and 125 µg per 100 mg of collagenous matrix as carrier (Fig. 4A), yielding corticalized ossicles by day 90 and expressing mRNA of bone induction markers such as BMP-3 and OP-1 [9]. The rapid architectural sculpture of mineralized constructs in the *rectus abdominis* by TGF-β isoforms solo or in binary application with hOP-1, a synergistic strategy known to yield massive ossicles in heterotopic sites, is a novel source of developing autoinduced bone for autogenous transplantation in clinical contexts.

The presence of several related but different molecular forms with osteogenic activity poses important questions about the biologic significance of this apparent redundancy, which also indicates multiple interactions during embryonic development and bone regeneration in postnatal life. The fact that a single recombinant hBMP/OP initiates bone formation by induction does not preclude the requirements and interactions of other morphogens deployed synchronously and synergistically during the cascade of bone formation by induction, which may proceed via the combined action of several BMPs/OPs resident within the natural milieu of the extracellular matrix of bone [6,10,27]. It is likely that the endogenous mechanisms of bone repair and regeneration in postnatal life necessitate the deployment and concerted action of several of the BMPs/OPs resident within the natural milieu of the extracellular matrix of bone [10,28–30].

The presence of multiple molecular forms with bone inductive activity also points to synergistic interactions during endochondral bone formation. A potent and accelerated synergistic induction of endochondral bone formation was shown with the binary application of recombinant or naturally derived TGF-β1 with hOP-1, in

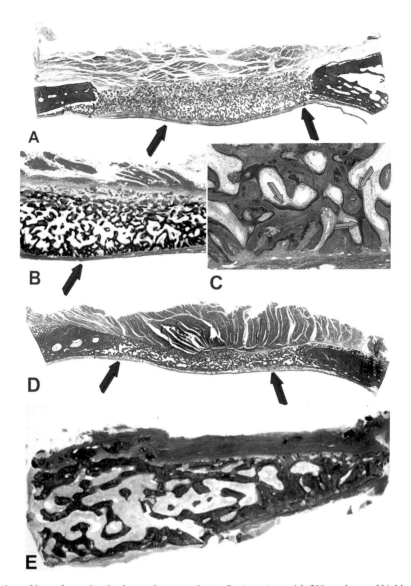

Fig. 2. Induction of bone formation in the nonhuman primate *Papio ursinus* with 280 μg doses of highly purified naturally derived BMPs/OPs, osteogenin, purified more than 70,000-fold from baboon demineralized and extracted bone matrices. (*A*) Defects in the calvarium of an adult baboon *Papio ursinus* show newly formed mineralized bone in blue resting on the dural layer (*blue arrows*) 30 days after application of the osteogenic proteins. (*B, C*) Higher power views highlight the newly formed mineralized bone surfaced by osteoid seams (*C, light blue arrows*) resting on the dural layer (*blue arrow*). (*D*) Complete regeneration of the calvarial defects 90 days after application of 280 μg of naturally derived partially purified osteogenic proteins. (*E*) Induction of bone formation after implantation of highly purified bovine BMPs/OPs in a mandibular defect of a human patient biopsied 90 days after implantation. Undecalcified sections cut at 5 μm stained free-floating with Goldner's trichrome. Original magnification: (*A*) ×2.5; (*B*) ×20; (*C*) ×90; (*D*) ×90.

heterotopic and orthotopic sites of primates (Fig. 4) [8–10].

Relatively low doses of DNA recombinantly produced or naturally derived TGF-β1 synergize with hOP-1 to induce massive heterotopic corticalized ossicles in the rectus abdominis muscle as early as 15 days after heterotopic implantation (Fig. 4C) and rapid and synergistic induction of

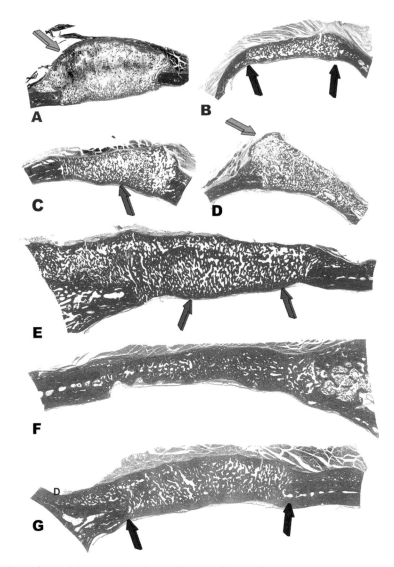

Fig. 3. Morphology of calvarial regeneration after application of doses of recombinant human osteogenic protein-1 delivered by bovine collagenous matrix making the hOP-1 osteogenic device. One gram of the device per calvarial defect. (*A, B*) Prominent osteogenesis on day 30 after application of 2.5 mg hOP-1 per gram of matrix with vascular and mesenchymal cell invasion within the newly formed ossicle together with scattered remnants of the collagenous matrix as carrier. (*B*) Complete regeneration after implantation of 0.1 mg hOP-1 per gram of carrier 90 days after implantation. (*C, D*) Extensive bone deposition 90 days after implantation of doses of the 2.5 mg hOP-1 osteogenic device. (*E–G*) Complete regeneration and maintenance of the newly formed bone in defect implanted with 2.5, 0.5, and 2.5 mg of the hOP-1 osteogenic device, respectively, and harvested 1 year after implantation in calvarial defects. Undecalcified sections cut at 5 μm stained free-floating with Goldner's trichrome. Original magnification: (*A–G*) ×2.5.

bone formation in nonhealing calvarial defects in adult baboons (Fig. 4E, F) [8–10]. It was noteworthy that the extent of bone induction by single applications of hOP-1 was raised several times by the combined application of comparatively low doses of recombinant or platelet-derived TGF-β1 (0.5, 1.5, and 5 μg); hTGF-β1 by itself induces endochondral bone at 5 μg/100 mg of carrier matrix (Fig. 4A) [8]. The tissue generated by the combined application of hOP-1 and hTGF-β1 shows distinct morphologic differences when compared with hOP-1-treated specimens, with large zones of endochondral development and extensive bone marrow formation with optimal synergy at a ratio

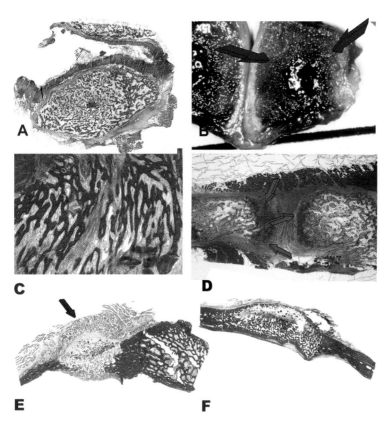

Fig. 4. Redundancy of soluble osteogenic molecular signals initiating bone formation in the rectus abdominis muscle of the nonhuman primate *Papio ursinus*. (*A*) Low power view of an ossicle induced after heterotopic extraskeletal implantation of 5 µg hTGF-β1delivered by 100 mg of allogeneic insoluble collagenous matrix as carrier. (*B*) Large corticalized ossicle harvested from the rectus abdominis muscle on day 15 after the synergistic interaction induced by binary applications of recombinant hOP-1 and hTGF-β1 in the rectus abdominis of an adult baboon. (*C*) Mineralized bone surfaced by osteoid seams populated by contiguous osteoblasts as early as 15 days after implantation by binary application of hOP-1 and relatively low doses of µg hTGF-β1. (*D*) Synergistic activity of doses of hOP-1 and hTGF-β1 resulting in the engineering of morphologic structures highly reminiscent of a rudimentary growth plate induced in the rectus abdominis muscle 30 days after implantation. (*E*) Prominent induction of bone formation in a calvarial defects 30 (*E*) and 90 (*F*) days after the binary application of 100 µg hOP-1 with 15 µg of naturally derived TGF-β1. Arrow indicates the pericranial growth of the newly induced bone. Undecalcified sections cut at 5 µm stained free-floating with Goldner's trichrome. Original magnification: (*A*) ×7.5; (*B*) ×2.5 (*C*) ×75; (*D*) ×3.5; (*E, F*) ×2.5.

of 20:1 by weight of hOP-1 and TGF-β1, respectively (Fig. 4H, G) [7,8].

The rapidity of tissue morphogenesis complete with mineralization of the outer cortex with bone marrow formation as early as 15 days after heterotopic implantation (Fig. 4B, C) bodes well for regeneration of bone in elderly persons, in whom repair phenomena are temporally delayed as compared with younger patients [8–10]. The binary applications of recombinant morphogens should result in novel synergistic molecular combinations for therapeutic osteogenesis in clinical contexts, obviating to the often limited bone induction by the single recombinant morphogen therapeutic approach.

Recapitulating development: a template for human osteoinduction

The replacement of missing bone is a major preoccupation of maxillofacial surgeons, and although the problem is often adequately solved with autologous bone grafts, the disadvantages associated with these procedures are considerable. In particular the challenges of large defects and defects in hypocellular sites are inadequately dealt with by autologous bone grafts. The considerable problem of donor site morbidity is a persistent accompaniment to the harvesting of bone grafts. Osteoinduction can be achieved in osseous (orthotopic) and nonosseous sites (heterotopic).

Clinically significant induction requires a recipient site of adequate cellularity to provide osteocompetent cells to respond to the molecular promptings of the implanted morphogens. Orthotopic application of an inductive device is limited to sites that are expected to be adequately vascularized. A bed that is highly vascular (ie, with minimal scarring) is necessary for orthotopic application, which should be reserved to sites that have been subjected to minimal previous surgery or radiation. Alternatively, all scar tissue must be removed meticulously to produce a recipient bed with multiple exposed vessels.

Several factors need careful consideration when developing an implantation algorithm for an inductive device. First, the choice of delivery system is influenced predominantly by the size and nature of the defect to be reconstructed. It should be carvable to allow adaptation to any defect morphology and be available in block and particulate forms. It should elicit no foreign body immune response and provide adequate structural support for load-bearing defects. Finally, it should be resorbable at a rate commensurate with the deposition and mineralization of new bone. To this end, several options are available (demineralized bone and bovine bone matrix, collagen sponge, resorbable synthetic polymers, synthetic hydroxyapatites) to the skeletal reconstructionist, none of which meets the aforementioned requirements. Clinicians must accept some compromises when making a choice, depending on the requirements of the particular defect that is to be repaired.

The delivery system also plays the significant role of temporal control of morphogen release. At this stage our understanding of morphogen desorption from different vehicles is incomplete, and close temporal control over morphogen release is currently impossible. Although it is clear that bone induction cascades occur because of the expression of protein morphogen at different times and sites, the recapitulation of this complexity is unachievable but fortunately may not be necessary. Future improvements in desorption control may optimize morphogen performance, particularly if multiple growth factors are being delivered.

The second major consideration is the choice of morphogen. The members of the TGF-β superfamily are constantly increasing, and to the consternation of the clinician-scientist many of them induce bone formation when singly applied. As far as morphogen selection is concerned, there are two broad choices: native (ie, extracted from bone) or recombinantly prepared. The major advantage of native BMP is that the extract is a heterogenous combination of several BMPs, which logically replicates the dosages and ratios in normal bone. Although there may be performance advantages for therapeutic application, standardization of isoform content and the ratios thereof is impossible and interpatient variability in results is to be expected. (Attempts to circumvent this result by in vivo batch testing in murine models are of little value because its significance for humans is doubtful.) Native BMP is not commercially available. Recombinant proteins can have the advantage of being produced homogenously and dosage can be reproduced accurately. Recombinant proteins are not subject to the theoretical disadvantage of disease transmission that naturally derived BMPs have.

The third consideration is the vexing question of how much morphogen? Development of dosage strategies has been extrapolated from animal data, which may not be of much value. Doses of single morphogen required for clinically significant osteoinduction are in the milligram range—massive in biologic terms. The only two recombinant morphogens commercially available are hOP-1 and hBMP-2, and clinicians are obliged to be pragmatic when selecting a recombinant morphogen rather than basing a decision on performance or application differentials.

To date, bone repair has been approached in a rather crude single morphogen approach and has resulted in uninspiring clinical performance at massive (and expensive) doses. The biologic evidence has demonstrated the benefits of multiple growth factors to massively improve osteoinductive performance at comparable doses. Bone formation (whether during development or for fracture repair) is the result of the concerted effects of many members of the TGF-β superfamily. The application of a single morphogen incompletely harnesses the biologic machinery for bone generation and the requirements of mega doses of morphogen to repair skeletal defects (which far exceed the total amount of protein present in the entire human skeleton). If nature can induce bone (and lots of it) with morphogen concentrations in the nanogram range and we require several milligrams to repair a relatively small defect, evidently something is amiss. Reassuringly adverse events thus far have not been reported after the use of recombinant OP-1 and BMP-2.

In cases in which orthotopic implantation is deemed unlikely to succeed, exploitation of distant, nonosseous, healthy body (heterotopic) sites as bone bioreactors allows the manufacture of prefabricated autologous transplants. The principal exploits myogenous sites, which are highly favorable for bone induction to occur. In humans, there are four published cases of prefabricated bone grafts replacing segments of the skeleton, all in the craniomaxillofacial skeleton (Fig. 5).

These techniques are not yet routinely used clinically because of unexpected inability to induce clinically significant bone in human patients.

Challenges in tissue engineering of bone: self-inducing biomimetic matrices and the induction of bone formation

The emergence in postnatal life of complex tissue morphologies rests on a simple and

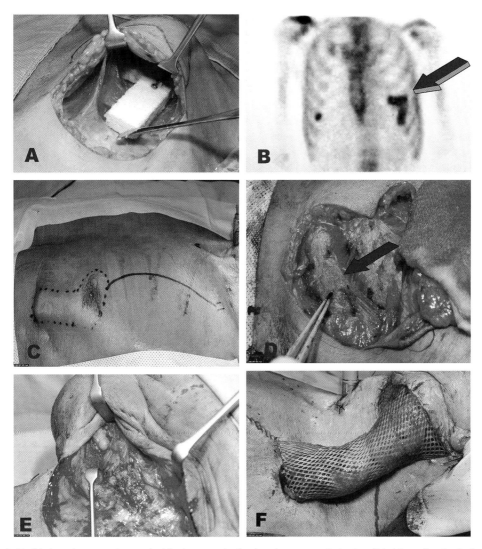

Fig. 5. Prefabricated osteogenic protein-1/hydroxyapatite implant into a vascularized pedicled bone flap in the human chest. (*A*) Surgical insertion of blocks of L-shaped porous hydroxyapatite preloaded with recombinant human osteogenic protein-1 into the left pectoralis major muscle of a human patient. (*B*) Skeletal scintigraphy demonstrates osteogenesis in the L-shaped chest implant. (*C*) Surgical preparation of the chest for the preparation of a pectoralis major myo-osseous–hydroxyapatite flap pedicled on the thoracoacromial artery. (*D*) Surgical débridement of the newly formed mandible (*arrow*). (*E*) Preparation of the recipient mandibular bed. (*F*) Placement of the pedicled flap in the left mandibular region.

fascinating concept: morphogens exploited in embryonic development are re-exploited and re-deployed to engineer tissue regeneration of postnatal tissues [1,3]. Embryonic development and tissue regeneration are equally regulated by selected few and highly conserved family of morphogens, members of the TGF-β supergene family [1,3].

The greatest challenge of regenerative medicine and tissue engineering of bone is translating in clinical contexts what has been so dramatically discovered in recent research studies [1,3,30]. Major fundamental research has made possible the emergence of tissue engineering to construct new tissues to restore impaired organs and regenerate lost parts of the human body [31]. The analysis of the molecular signals in solution has led to the understanding of the mechanisms of cell differentiation, development, and morphogenesis and the emerging science of tissue engineering and regenerative medicine [1,3–5]. Perhaps the greatest advance of all has been the understanding that postnatal tissue regeneration and regenerative medicine and tissue engineering are recapitulations of embryonic development [1,3]. The families of the BMPs/OPs and TGF-β proteins are an elegant example of nature's parsimony in programming multiple specialized functions or pleiotropy [1,3]. BMPs/OPs and TGF-βs uniquely in primates induce postnatal de novo endochondral bone formation as a recapitulation of embryonic development and act as soluble signals of tissue morphogenesis sculpting the multicellular mineralized structures of the bone/bone marrow organ [1,3–5]. The postnatal induction of heterotopic bone rests on a simple and fascinating concept: morphogens exploited in embryonic development can be re-exploited and redeployed to engineer tissue regeneration of postnatal tissues [1,3,4]. We have learned that embryonic development and tissue regeneration are equally regulated by a few selected and highly conserved family of morphogens, members of the TGF-β supergene family [1,3,4].

Ultimately, predictable and optimal osteogenesis in clinical contexts requires information concerning the expression and cross-regulation of gene products of the osteogenic proteins of the TGF-β supergene family elicited by a single application of a recombinant morphogen [3,7]. Long-term experiments in the primate *Papio ursinus* have indicated a critical role of gamma-irradiated hOP-1 delivered by xenogeneic bovine collagenous bone matrices to completely regenerate and maintain the architecture of the induced bone after treatment of nonhealing calvarial defects with single applications of doses of 0.1, 0.5, and 2.5 mg hOP-1 per gram of xenogeneic matrix [6]. Northern blot analyses of total RNA generated from tissues induced by the hOP-1 osteogenic device in heterotopic and orthotopic calvarial sites have provided insights into the distinct spatial and temporal patterns of gene expression of members of the TGF-β superfamily, including OP-1, BMP-3, GDF-10, and TGF-β1 and collagen types II and IV [7]. High levels of expression of OP-1 mRNA demonstrate autoinduction of OP-1 mRNA during tissue induction by hOP-1 [7]. The temporal and spatial expression of TGF-β1 mRNA indicates a specific temporal window during which expression of TGF- β1 is mandatory for successful and optimal osteogenesis [7].

We have shown that the induction of bone formation can be restored by matrices other than the insoluble collagenous bone matrix, such as porous hydroxyapatite, as carrier in rodents and nonhuman primates (Fig. 6) [25,27].

These experiments have demonstrated clearly that the induction of the complex tissue morphologies of the bone/bone marrow organ and periodontal tissues develops as a mosaic structure in which the osteogenic proteins of the TGF-β supergene family singly, synergistically, and synchronously initiate and maintain tissue induction and morphogenesis [3–7]. The presence of multiple molecular forms with bone inductive activity points to several complex synergistic interactions during bone formation by induction [3]. Binary applications of recombinant hOP-1 and relatively low doses of hTGF-β1 synergize in inducing massive ossicles in heterotopic and orthotopic sites of the baboon as early as 15 days after implantation [8,9]. Binary combinations should ow be used in humans to avoid supraphysiologic doses of single recombinant proteins as currently required in clinical contexts.

Perhaps the most elegant way to induce the heterotopic induction of bone formation is to create smart, self-inducing biomimetic matrices that are endowed with the striking prerogative of initiating de novo bone formation (Fig. 6D–G); they induce new bone formation even if implanted in extraskeletal heterotopic sites without the addition of exogenously applied BMPs/OPs (Fig. 7) [25,32,33]. Regenerative medicine and tissue engineering of bone start by erecting scaffolds of biomimetic biomaterial matrices that mimic the

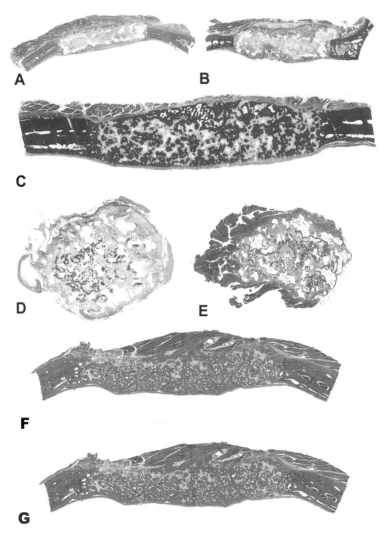

Fig. 6. Morphology of calvarial repair 30 days after implantation of porous sintered crystalline hydroxyapatites pre-loaded with 100 (*A*) and 500 (*B*) μg hOP-1. (*C*) Calvarial repair after implantation of a porous sintered crystalline hydroxyapatite and 500 μg hOP-1 harvested on day 90. (*D, E*) Morphogenesis of bone in porous sintered crystalline hydroxyapatite 90 days after implantation within the rectus abdominis muscle and without the exogenous application of BMPs/OPs. (*F, G*) Complete induction of bone formation across the porous spaces of crystalline hydroxyapatite biomatrices harvested from calvarial defects 90 days after implantation without the exogenous application of BMPs/OPs.

supramolecular assembly of the extracellular matrix of bone [25,32,33].

The complex cellular, molecular, and mechanical signals that regulate the assembly of the extracellular matrix precisely regulate angiogenesis and vascular invasion [3]. The instructive role of the extracellular matrix via affinity of amino acid sequences interacting with molecular signals of the TGF-β superfamily results in tissue patterning in embryonic development and is recapitulated and redeployed postnatally for the induction and

morphogenesis of the bone/bone-marrow organ [1,5,7,8].

The conceptual framework of tissue induction and regeneration would not be possible without the knowledge of the binding and sequestration of angiogenic and osteogenic proteins that provide the conceptual framework of the supramolecular assembly of the extracellular matrix of bone [1, 3–5]. Angiogenic and bone morphogenetic proteins bound to type IV collagen of the invading capillaries are presented in an immobilized form

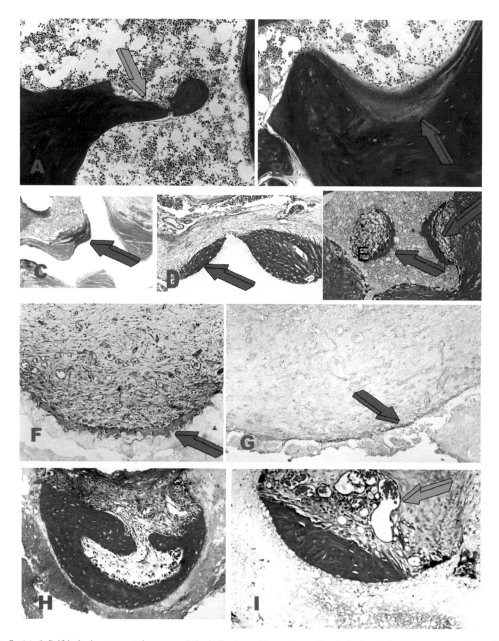

Fig. 7. (*A–I*) Self-inducing geometric cues and the induction of bone formation in heterotopic intramuscular sites of the baboon. Angiogenesis and capillary invasion (*arrows*) within the soft tissues invading the concavity of a hydroxyapatite biomimetic matrix 90 days after implantation in the rectus abdominis muscle. Induced capillaries face the induction of bone that had formed within the concavity of the biomimetic matrix. Decalcified matrix cut at 5 μm. Original magnification: ×75.

to responding mesenchymal cells to initiate osteogenesis in angiogenesis [1,3,5,11]. By sequestering initiators and promoters of angiogenesis and bone morphogenesis, basement membrane components are modeling bone formation by induction in angiogenesis [3–5].

Bone formation by induction initiates by invocation of soluble molecular signals that combined with insoluble signals or substrata trigger the ripple-like cascade of cell differentiation into osteoblastic cells lines that secrete bone matrix at the site of surgical implantation [1,3]. A most exciting and novel strategy for initiating bone formation by induction is carving smart, self-inducing geometric concavities assembled within biomimetic matrices endowed with the striking prerogative of differentiating osteoblastic-like cells attached to the concavities secreting bone matrix without the exogenous application of soluble osteogenic molecular signals of the TGF-β superfamily (Fig. 7) [3,32,33]. Expression of mRNA species is followed by secretion and embedding of the expressed gene products into the concavities (Fig. 7G), which results in secondary induction of bone formation in angiogenesis (Fig. 7H, I) [4,33].

The intrinsic induction of bone formation is a relatively novel and cost-effective bone tissue engineering strategy based on the expression and secretion of osteogenic molecular signals as initiated by geometrically smart, self-inducing matrices (Fig. 7) [3,32,33]. Independently, other research groups reported the induction of bone formation in various phosphate ceramics in different animal models, including sheep [34,35]. This finding is a fascinating phenomenon—that is, biomimetic biomaterial matrices that arouse and set into motion the mammalian body's natural ability to heal and construct biomimetic matrices, which in their own right set into motion inductive regenerative phenomena that initiate the cascade of bone differentiation by induction [3,32,33].

The induction of bone formation by smart biomimetic matrices with a series of repetitive concavities that initiate bone differentiation by induction is also a recapitulation of the remodeling cycle of the osteonic bone, in which concavities as induced by osteoclastogenesis (Fig. 7A) are filled with newly formed bone or osteoid recapitulating the phenomena of bone formation by induction within the concavities of the biomimetic biomaterial matrices.

Major research efforts should be devoted to the construction of biomimetic biomaterial matrices self-inducing osteogenesis in angiogenesis without the addition of soluble osteogenic molecular signals of the TGF-β superfamily. This is a most exciting way to initiate bone formation by induction, (ie, mimic the supersmart functionalities of living tissues by providing biomimetic matrices that are endowed with the striking prerogative of initiating bone formation by induction, even if the biomimetic matrices are implanted in heterotopic extraskeletal sites without the addition of exogenously applied osteogenic molecular signals of the TGF-β superfamily) [3–5].

A word of caution: scientifically, major interdisciplinary efforts of molecular cellular and developmental biology and experimental surgery have led scientists and surgeons to believe that novel tissue engineering strategies are available to improve human life, lengthen lifespan, and keep humans functional as long as possible by using regenerative medicine [36,37]. Humans are living longer and aspiring to a higher quality of life into an advanced age [30,36]. The translation of tissue engineering strategies as achieved in animal models has been hampered by several problems and limitations, however, not the least of which is that research in human patients has dramatically shown that the induction of bone is on a different scale altogether when compared with animals models, including nonhuman primates. Although tissue engineering is a field of tremendous promise, novel methods dramatically shown in animal models, are not yet applicable to routine clinical applications and commercial production, although they occasionally are applied with success in humans [30,38]. Ultimately, it is still doubtful whether tissue engineering will emerge as a winning medical technology or fail [30].

Economies must change and change globally to allow tissue-engineered constructs to be routinely deployed in clinical contexts [30,36,38]. Although regenerative medicine and tissue engineering are able—at least in experimental animals—to implement regenerative procedures effectively, technologies required to implement tissue-engineered constructs (including the creation of ex vivo or in vivo tissues such as bone for mandibular reconstruction) are still sophisticated and specialized technologies that may cause further inequalities in different populations around the globe. An incisive contribution by Williams [30] provided important perspectives on tissue engineering faced by the twenty-first century and placed the well-funded hopes and despair of clinical and commercial reality on a balanced scientific foundation [30].

The emerging science of tissue engineering has facilitated dramatically our understanding of the biochemical and molecular mechanisms of growth and differentiation, development, and morphogenesis and has induced the regeneration of tissues lost as a consequence of trauma and disease [30,31]. Regretfully, however, regenerative medicine and tissue engineering have the potential to further enhance the iniquities and inequalities among humans on planet Earth, with the potential for a dramatic impact on national economies [36].

By deploying the osteogenic soluble molecular signals combined with selected substrata or insoluble signals, however, regenerative medicine and tissue engineering have made possible novel regenerative strategies for the reconstruction of bone in humans [39,40] and the generation of bone bioreactors for in vivo tissue engineering of organs [39–41].

The basic tissue engineering paradigm is tissue and organ development and morphogenesis by combining soluble signals and insoluble substrata in the presence of viable responding cells [1,3] acting as a three-dimensional scaffold for the initiation of de novo tissue induction and morphogenesis [1]. The induction of bone formation, by combining soluble signals of the TGF-β superfamily with various carriers delivering the osteogenic activity at site of surgical implantation, is the essence of the tissue-engineering paradigm so that tissue engineering is still learning the secrets of its principles from the induction of bone formation by the soluble osteogenic molecular signals of the TGF-β superfamily [1]. Soluble and insoluble signals and responding cells mechanistically trigger the cascade of bone tissue engineering as a recapitulation of embryonic development [1–5].

Significant for all tissue engineering strategies is our knowledge that the extracellular matrix is the scaffold that binds and releases soluble molecular signals, sequesters them in the solid state, and presents them in the right conformation to ligands on responding cells. Only time will tell, however, if the tissue-engineering paradigm will be used routinely in clinical contexts and if the fundamental major discoveries in molecular and cellular biology and experimental surgery that have led to the emerging science of regenerative medicine can be rigorously adopted to the challenge of fabricating new tissues and organs of the human body [30].

Acknowledgments

Supported by the SA MRC, the University of the Witwatersrand, Johannesburg and the National Research Foundation. The authors thank Barbara van den Heever, June Teare, Louise Renton, and Ruqayya Parak for the unique undecalcified sections of bone and the Central Animal Services of the University for the help with primate experimentation. The authors also thank M. Thomas, W. Richter and the Council for Scientific and Industrial Research, Pretoria, for the preparation of the biomimetic matrices for heterotopic and orthotopic implanation.

References

[1] Reddi AH. Morphogenesis and tissue engineering of bone and cartilage: inductive signals, stem cells, and biomimetic biomaterials. Tissue Eng 2000;6:351–9.

[2] Wozney JM. The bone morphogenetic protein family and osteogenesis. Mol Reprod Dev 1992;32:160–7.

[3] Ripamonti U. Soluble osteogenic molecular signals and the induction of bone formation. Biomaterials 2006;27:807–22.

[4] Ripamonti U. Embedding molecular signals in biomimetic matrices for regenerative medicine. S Afr J Sci 2006;102:211–6.

[5] Ripamonti U, Herbst NN, Ramoshebi LN. Bone morphogenetic proteins in craniofacial and periodontal tissue engineering: experimental studies in the non-human primate Papio ursinus. Cytokine Growth Factor Rev 2005;16:357–68.

[6] Ripamonti U, van den Heever B, Crooks J, et al. Long-term evaluation of bone formation by osteogenic protein-1 in the baboon and relative efficacy of bone-derived bone morphogenetic proteins delivered by irradiated xenogeneic collagenous matrices. J Bone Miner Res 2000;15:1798–809.

[7] Ripamonti U. Bone induction by recombinant human osteogenic protein-1 (hOP-1, BMP-7) in the primate Papio ursinus with expression of mRNA of gene products of the TGF-ß superfamily. J Cell Mol Med 2005;9:911–28.

[8] Ripamonti U, Duneas N, van den Heever B, et al. Recombinant transforming growth factor-β1 induces endochondral bone in the baboon and synergizes with recombinant osteogenic protein-1 (bone morphogenetic protein-7) to initiate rapid bone formation. J Bone Miner Res 1997;2:1584–95.

[9] Duneas N, Crooks J, Ripamonti U. Transforming growth factor-β1: induction of bone morphogenetic protein genes expression during endochondral bone formation in the baboon, and synergistic interaction with osteogenic protein-1 (BMP-7). Growth Factors 1998;15:259–77.

[10] Ripamonti U. Osteogenic proteins of the TGF-β superfamily. In: Henry HL, Norman AW, editors. Encyclopedia of hormones. San Diego (CA): Austin Academic Press; 2003. p. 80–6.

[11] Ripamonti U, Ferretti C, Heliotis M. Soluble and insoluble signals and the induction of bone formation: molecular therapeutics recapitulating development. J Anat 2006;209:447–68.

[12] Spemann H. Embryonic development and induction. New Haven (CT): Yale University Press; 1938.

[13] Levander G. Tissue induction. Nature 1945;155:148–9.

[14] Urist MR. Bone: formation by autoinduction. Science 1965;150:893–9.

[15] Turing AM. The chemical basis of morphogenesis. Philos Trans R Soc Lond 1952;45B:402–18.

[16] Ripamonti U, Duneas N. Tissue morphogenesis and regeneration by bone morphogeneteic proteins. Plast Recontsr Surg 1998;101:227–39.

[17] Sampath TK, Reddi AH. Dissociative extraction and reconstitution of extracellular matrix components involved in local bone differentiation. Proc Natl Acad Sci U S A 1981;78:7599–603.

[18] Urist MR, Huo YK, Brownell AG, et al. Purification of bovine bone morphogenetic protein by hydroxyapatite chromatography. Proc Natl Acad Sci U S A 1984;81:371–5.

[19] Wang EA, Rosen V, Cordes P, et al. Purification and characterization of other distinct bone-inducing factors. Proc Natl Acad Sci U S A 1988;85:9484–8.

[20] Luyten FP, Cunningham NS, Ma S, et al. Purification and partial amino-acid sequence of osteogenin, a protein initiating bone differentiation. J Biolumin Chemilumin 1998;264:13377–80.

[21] Ripamonti U, Ma S, Cunningham N, et al. Initiation of bone regeneration in adult baboons by osteogenin, a bone morphogenetic protein. Matrix 1992; 12:369–80.

[22] Sampath TK, Reddi AH. Homology of bone-inductive proteins from human, monkey, bovine and rat extracellular matrix. Proc Natl Acad Sci U S A 1983;80:6591–695.

[23] Ripamonti U, Reddi AH. Bone morphogenetic proteins: applications in plastic and reconstructive surgery. Adv Plast Reconstr Surg 1995;11:47–73.

[24] Wozney JM, Rosen V, Celeste AJ, et al. Novel regulators of bone formation: molecular clones and activities. Science 1988;242:1528–34.

[25] Ripamonti U, Ramoshebi LN, Matsaba T, et al. Bone induction by BMPs/OPs and related family members in primates: the critical role of delivery systems. J Bone Joint Surg 2001;83-A(Suppl 1):116–27.

[26] Roberts AB, Sporn MB, Assoian RK, et al. Transforming growth factor type β: rapid induction of fibrosis and angiogenesis in vivo and stimulation of collagen formation in vitro. Proc Natl Acad Sci U S A 1986;83:4167–71.

[27] Ripamonti U, Ramoshebi LN, Patton J, et al. Soluble signals and insoluble substrata: novel molecular cues instructing the induction of bone. In: Massaro EJ, Rogers JM, editors. The skeleton. Totowa (NJ): Humana Press; 2004. p. 217.

[28] Orringer JS, Shaw WW, Borud LJ, et al. Total mandibular and lower lip reconstruction with a prefabricated osteocutaneous free flap. Plast Reconstr Surg 1999;104:793–7.

[29] Arnander C, Westermark A, Veltheim R, et al. Three-dimensional technology and bone morphogenetic protein in frontal bone reconstruction. J Craniofac Surg 2006;17:275–9.

[30] Williams DF. Tissue engineering: the multidisciplinary epitome of hope and despair. In: Paton R, McNamara L, editors. Studies in multidisciplinarity. Elsevier BV; 2006. p. 483–524.

[31] Reddi AH. Role of morphogenetic proteins in skeletal tissue engineering and regeneration. Nat Biotechnol 1998;16:247–52.

[32] Ripamonti U, Crooks J, Kirkbride AN. Sintered porous hydroxyapatites with intrinsic osteoinductive activity: geometric induction of bone formation. S Afr J Sci 1999;95:335–43.

[33] Ripamonti U. Self-inducing shape memory geometric cues embedded within smart hydroxyapatite-based biomimetic matrices. Plast Reconstr Surg, in press.

[34] Yuan H, van Blitterswijk CA, de Groot K, et al. Cross-species comparison of ectopic bone formation in biphasic calcium phosphate (BCP) and hydroxyapatite (HA) scaffolds. Tissue Eng 2006;12: 1607–15.

[35] Gosain AK, Song L, Riordan P, et al. A 1-year study of osteoinduction in hydroxyapatite-derived biomaterials in an adult sheep model: Part I. Plast Reconstr Surg 2002;109:619–30.

[36] Stupp SI. Biomaterials for regenerative medicine. MRS Bull 2005;30:546–53.

[37] Vacanti CA. The history of tissue engineering. J Cell Mol Med 2006;10:569–76.

[38] Mansbridge J. Commercial considerations in tissue engineering. J Anat 2006;209:527–32.

[39] Warnke PH, Springer ING, Wiltfang J, et al. Growth and transplantation of a custom vascularised bone graft in a man. Lancet 2004;364: 766–70.

[40] Heliotis M, Lavery KM, Ripamonti U, et al. Transformation of a prefabricated hydroxyapatite/osteogenic protein-1 implant into a vascularised pedicled bone flap in the human chest. Int J Oral Maxillofac Surg 2006;35:265–9.

[41] Stevens MM, Marini RP, Schaefer D, et al. In vivo engineering of organs: the bone bioreactor. Proc Natl Acad Sci U S A 2005;102:11450–5.

ELSEVIER
SAUNDERS

Oral Maxillofacial Surg Clin N Am 19 (2007) 591–595

ORAL AND
MAXILLOFACIAL
SURGERY CLINICS
of North America

Index

Note: Page numbers of article titles are in **boldface** type.

United States Postal Service

Statement of Ownership, Management, and Circulation
(All Periodicals Publications Except Requestor Publications)

1. Publication Title
Oral and Maxillofacial Surgery Clinics of North America

2. Publication Number
0 0 6 - 3 6 2

3. Filing Date
9/14/07

4. Issue Frequency
Feb, May, Aug, Nov

5. Number of Issues Published Annually
4

6. Annual Subscription Price
$218.00

7. Complete Mailing Address of Known Office of Publication (Not printer) (Street, city, county, state, and ZIP+4)
Elsevier Inc.
360 Park Avenue South
New York, NY 10010-1710

Contact Person
Stephen Bushing

Telephone (Include area code)
215-239-3688

8. Complete Mailing Address of Headquarters or General Business Office of Publisher (Not printer)
Elsevier Inc., 360 Park Avenue South, New York, NY 10010-1710

9. Full Names and Complete Mailing Addresses of Publisher, Editor, and Managing Editor (Do not leave blank)

Publisher (Name and complete mailing address)
John Schrefer, Elsevier, Inc., 1600 John F. Kennedy Blvd. Suite 1800, Philadelphia, PA 19103-2899

Editor (Name and complete mailing address)
John Vassallo, Elsevier, Inc., 1600 John F. Kennedy Blvd. Suite 1800, Philadelphia, PA 19103-2899

Managing Editor (Name and complete mailing address)
Catherine Bewick, Elsevier, Inc., 1600 John F. Kennedy Blvd. Suite 1800, Philadelphia, PA 19103-2899

10. Owner (Do not leave blank. If the publication is owned by a corporation, give the name and address of the corporation immediately followed by the names and addresses of all stockholders owning or holding 1 percent or more of the total amount of stock. If not owned by a corporation, give the names and addresses of the individual owners. If owned by a partnership or other unincorporated firm, give its name and address as well as those of each individual owner. If the publication is published by a nonprofit organization, give its name and address.)

Full Name	Complete Mailing Address
Wholly owned subsidiary of	4520 East-West Highway
Reed/Elsevier, US holdings	Bethesda, MD 20814

11. Known Bondholders, Mortgagees, and Other Security Holders Owning or Holding 1 Percent or More of Total Amount of Bonds, Mortgages, or Other Securities. If none, check box → None

Full Name	Complete Mailing Address
N/A	

12. Tax Status (For completion by nonprofit organizations authorized to mail at nonprofit rates) (Check one)
The purpose, function, and nonprofit status of this organization and the exempt status for federal income tax purposes:
☐ Has Not Changed During Preceding 12 Months
☐ Has Changed During Preceding 12 Months (Publisher must submit explanation of change with this statement)

13. Publication Title
Oral and Maxillofacial Surgery Clinics of North America

14. Issue Date for Circulation Data Below
May 2007

15. Extent and Nature of Circulation

		Average No. Copies Each Issue During Preceding 12 Months	No. Copies of Single Issue Published Nearest to Filing Date
a. Total Number of Copies (Net press run)		3300	3400
b. Paid Circulation (By Mail and Outside the Mail)	(1) Mailed Outside-County Paid Subscriptions Stated on PS Form 3541. (Include paid distribution above nominal rate, advertiser's proof copies, and exchange copies)	2095	2071
	(2) Mailed In-County Paid Subscriptions Stated on PS Form 3541 (Include paid distribution above nominal rate, advertiser's proof copies, and exchange copies)		
	(3) Paid Distribution Outside the Mails Including Sales Through Dealers and Carriers, Street Vendors, Counter Sales, and Other Paid Distribution Outside USPS®	340	329
	(4) Paid Distribution by Other Classes Mailed Through the USPS (e.g. First-Class Mail®)		
c. Total Paid Distribution (Sum of 15b (1), (2), (3), and (4))		2435	2400
d. Free or Nominal Rate Distribution (By Mail and Outside the Mail)	(1) Free or Nominal Rate Outside-County Copies Included on PS Form 3541	213	186
	(2) Free or Nominal Rate In-County Copies Included on PS Form 3541		
	(3) Free or Nominal Rate Copies Mailed at Other Classes Mailed Through the USPS (e.g. First-Class Mail)		
	(4) Free or Nominal Rate Distribution Outside the Mail (Carriers or other means)		
e. Total Free or Nominal Rate Distribution (Sum of 15d (1), (2), (3) and (4))		213	186
f. Total Distribution (Sum of 15c and 15e)		2648	2586
g. Copies not Distributed (See instructions to publishers #4 (page #3))		652	814
h. Total (Sum of 15f and g)		3300	3400
i. Percent Paid (15c divided by 15f times 100)		91.96%	92.81%

16. Publication of Statement of Ownership
☐ If the publication is a general publication, publication of this statement is required. Will be printed in the November 2007 issue of this publication. ☐ Publication not required

17. Signature and Title of Editor, Publisher, Business Manager, or Owner

[signature] Stephen Bushing – Executive Director of Subscription Services

Date: September 14, 2007

I certify that all information furnished on this form is true and complete. I understand that anyone who furnishes false or misleading information on this form or who omits material or information requested on the form may be subject to criminal sanctions (including fines and imprisonment) and/or civil sanctions (including civil penalties).

PS Form 3526, September 2006 (Page 2 of 3)

PS Form 3526, September 2006 (Page 1 of 3 (Instructions Page 3)) PSN 7530-01-000-9931 PRIVACY NOTICE: See our Privacy policy in www.usps.com

SPACE MATH

By Amanda Onion

CELEBRATION PRESS

Pearson Learning Group

The following people from **Pearson Learning Group**
have contributed to the development of this product:

Design Tricia Battipede, Evelyn Bauer, Bernadette Hruby, Jennifer Visco
Marketing Kimberly Doster, Gina Konopinski-Jacobia
Editorial Leslie Feierstone Barna, Madeline Boskey Olsen, Jennifer Van Der Heide
Production Irene Belinsky, Mark Cirillo, Roxanne Knoll, Ruth Leine, Susan Levine
Visual Acquisitions Mindy Klarman, David Mager, Judy Mahoney, Salita Mehta, Elbaliz Mendez, Alison O'Brien, Dan Thomas
Content Area Consultant Mary Ann Zagar

The following people from **DK**
have contributed to the development of this product:

Managing Art Director Richard Czapnik
Project Manager Nigel Duffield
Editorial Lead Heather Jones
Design Ann Cannings

All photography © Pearson Education, Inc. (PEI) unless otherwise specifically noted.

Photographs: Cover: *t.* NASA/Johnson Space Center; *b.* NASA/John F. Kennedy Space Center. Back Cover: NASA/Johnson Space Center. 1: NASA Headquarters. 1–32: border NASA Headquarters. 3: David Nunuk/Photo Researchers, Inc. 4: *l.* Novastock/The Stock Connection; *r.* Raymond Gehman/National Geographic Society. 5: NASA/DK Images. 6: David R. Frazier/Photo Researchers, Inc. 7: NASA/Johnson Space Center. 8: U.S. Department of Defense. 9: NASA Headquarters. 10: *m.r.* Tim Ridley © DK Images; *b.r.* Tim Ridley © DK Images. 11: *l.* Mike Dunning/Peter Griffiths—modelmaker © DK Images; *m.* NASA/DK Images; *r.* © DK Images. 12–13: NASA Headquarters. 13: NASA. 14–15: NASA/John F. Kennedy Space Center. 16: NASA/Finley Holiday Films/DK Images. 17: bkgd. © Bettmann/Corbis; *l. to r. insets* Julian Baum © DK Images, NASA/DK Images, NASA/DK Images, Julian Baum © DK Images, Julian Baum © DK Images, NASA/DK Images, JPL/DK Images, NASA/Finley Holiday Films/DK Images. 18: Omni-Photo Communications, Inc. 19: NASA/Johnson Space Center. 20–21: Southern Stock/Index Stock Imagery, Inc. 22–23: NASA/Johnson Space Center. 24: © Michael Kim/Corbis. 25: © Reuters/Corbis. 26: © Reuters/Corbis. 27: AFP/Getty Images, Inc. 28: SPL/Photo Researchers, Inc. 29: Chris Cook/Photo Researchers, Inc. 30: John R. Foster/Photo Researchers, Inc. 32: David A. Wagner/Phototake.

ISBN-13: 978-0-7652-8634-5

ISBN-10:   0-7652-8634-3

Printed in the United States of America
1 2 3 4 5 6 7 8 9 10   11 10 09 08 07

1-800-321-3106
www.pearsonlearning.com

Contents

Big Space

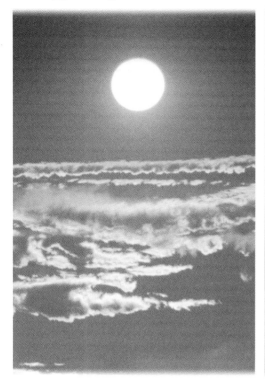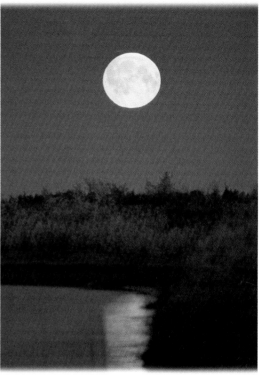

The Sun and Moon look similar in size when viewed from Earth.

Space is a big place. It is such a big place that it takes math to understand it. Scientists use math to measure distances in space. They use math to learn how fast objects in space move and how big they are.

The Sun and Moon sometimes appear to be the same size in the sky. In fact, however, millions of moons would fit inside the Sun. Why do they appear to be the same size? It is because the Sun is much farther away from us than the Moon. The farther away an object is, the smaller it appears.

Scientists use math every time they want to do something in space. For example, when scientists carry out a space shuttle launch, it takes math to get the shuttle into space. It also takes math to get the shuttle to its destination. Every bit of planning in a space mission requires math. In this book, you'll learn about some of the math that scientists use to explore space.

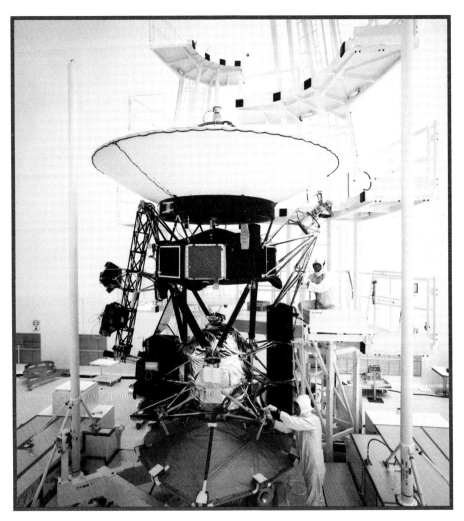

Space scientists use math to prepare a shuttle for a mission.

How Near? How Far?

When the Moon is full, it appears very big in the night sky. However, the planet Earth is actually four times larger in diameter than the Moon. The Moon appears to be so large because it is our closest neighbor in space. It is about 384,401 **kilometers** away. That's about 238,857 miles. To travel that distance on Earth, a person would have to circle Earth ten times.

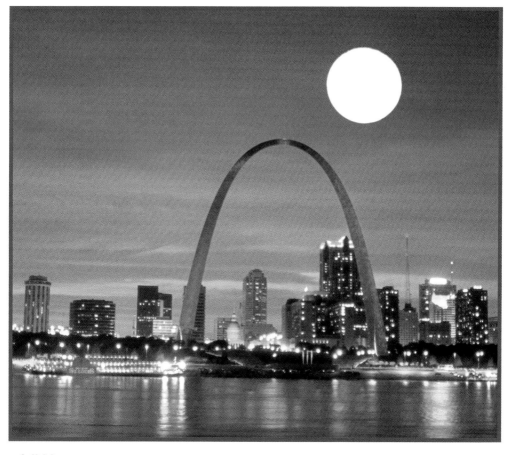

a full Moon

So how do scientists measure the distance to the Moon? It's much too far to use a tape measure. One way to estimate the distance to the Moon is by using **lasers**, which send out intense beams of light. When astronauts walked on the Moon during a space mission, they left behind four mirrors. The mirrors are each about the size of a computer screen. By aiming lasers at these mirrors, scientists can measure the distance to the Moon.

The Earth and the Moon are neighbors.

Suppose that a person can walk 1 mile in 20 minutes. How far can that person walk in 1 hour? The answer is 3 miles, because 20 minutes times 3 miles is 60 minutes, or 1 hour. In the same way, scientists use light in their **calculations** of distance. Light moves faster than any other object in space. It travels at 186,000 miles per second!

The lasers' beams travel to the Moon and bounce off the mirrors. Then they return to Earth. The time it takes them to do this tells scientists how far the beams traveled. Using this math, scientists can **precisely** measure the distance between Earth and the Moon.

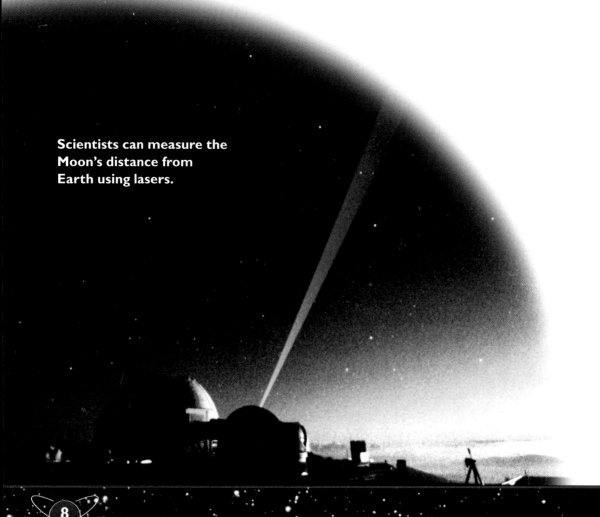

Scientists can measure the Moon's distance from Earth using lasers.

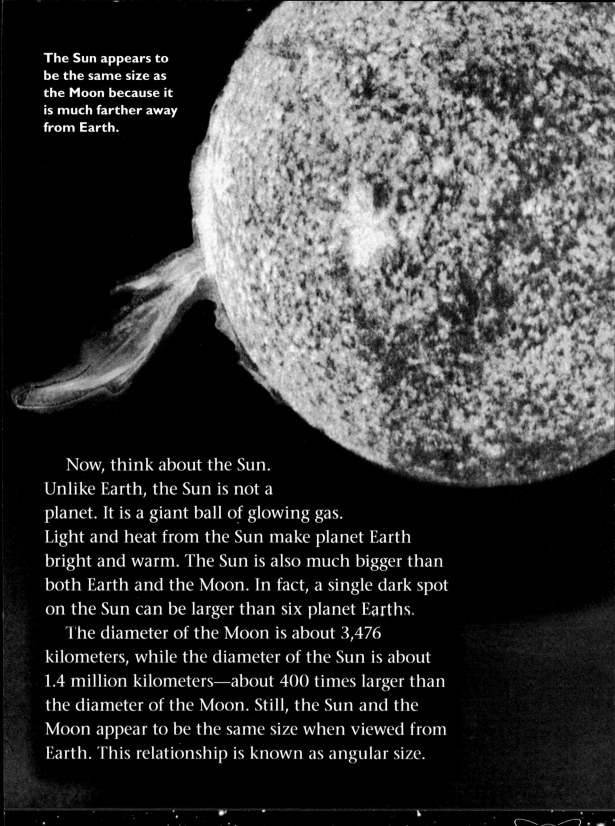

The Sun appears to be the same size as the Moon because it is much farther away from Earth.

Now, think about the Sun.
Unlike Earth, the Sun is not a
planet. It is a giant ball of glowing gas.
Light and heat from the Sun make planet Earth
bright and warm. The Sun is also much bigger than
both Earth and the Moon. In fact, a single dark spot
on the Sun can be larger than six planet Earths.

The diameter of the Moon is about 3,476
kilometers, while the diameter of the Sun is about
1.4 million kilometers—about 400 times larger than
the diameter of the Moon. Still, the Sun and the
Moon appear to be the same size when viewed from
Earth. This relationship is known as angular size.

Angular size is the apparent size of an object—or the way it appears. Angular size is measured in degrees, the way angles are measured. As an example, imagine looking at two balls of different sizes. A baseball is about three times bigger in diameter than a table tennis ball. The baseball looks bigger if you put them beside each other. Now imagine placing the baseball several feet away from the smaller ball. When a person looks at them this way using one eye, the balls seem the same size. This is the effect of angular size.

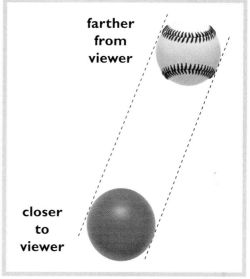

farther from viewer

closer to viewer

A baseball is larger than a table tennis ball, but they look the same size when the larger ball is placed behind the smaller one.

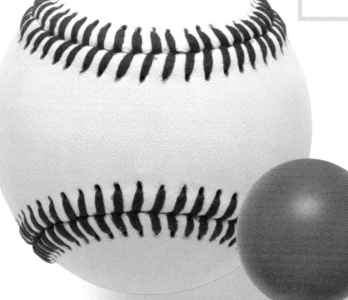

One effect of the Sun and the Moon having the same angular size is that a solar eclipse is possible. A solar eclipse occurs when the Moon travels between the Earth and the Sun, and it appears to cover the Sun nearly completely. When this happens, the Moon casts a shadow on parts of Earth. An eclipse can make it appear dark during the middle of the day.

Scientists use solar eclipses to make different calculations about space. More than 2,000 years ago, a Greek scientist used a solar eclipse to measure the distance to the Moon. The scientist, Hipparchus, measured how much of the Sun appeared behind the Moon during an eclipse as seen from two different points on Earth.

Hipparchus measured the angles formed by lines of sight from the two spots on Earth to the Moon and to the Sun. He used those measurements to calculate the distance of the Moon to Earth. As it turned out, the number he came up with was too large because he had assumed that the peak of the eclipse took place at exactly the same time at both points. Still, it's amazing that he was able to do this calculation 2,000 years ago—without the benefit of computers.

Solar Eclipse Geometry

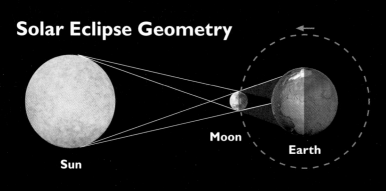

Sun

Moon

Earth

During a solar eclipse, the Moon moves between Earth and the Sun and casts a shadow.

Calculations Count!

Planning a space mission takes so many calculations that many people have to work on the plan at once. Working together gets the job done faster, but it also means scientists have to be sure they use the same kind of measurements—otherwise mistakes can happen. Nowhere is this fact more evident than in space exploration.

What sorts of calculations do astronauts do on a mission? They need to understand what the spacecraft is doing and how it operates.

For instance, when a satellite is released into orbit, astronauts use geometry to calculate the distance from the satellite to the shuttle. They use angles formed by their line of sight to the satellite.

Computers do the most difficult math on a mission. However, there are times when calculations done by hand are needed, as the history of the moon missions shows.

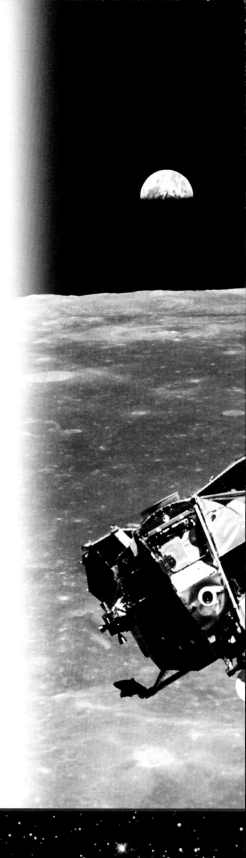

On July 16, 1969, during the first Apollo lunar-landing mission, two astronauts walked on the Moon. A third astronaut remained in the spacecraft, while Neil Armstrong and Edwin Aldrin Jr. spent 2½ hours on the surface of the Moon. The entire mission lasted 8 days, and the spacecraft landed safely in the Pacific Ocean, as planned.

Astronaut Neil Armstrong took this photograph of Edwin Aldrin on the Moon.

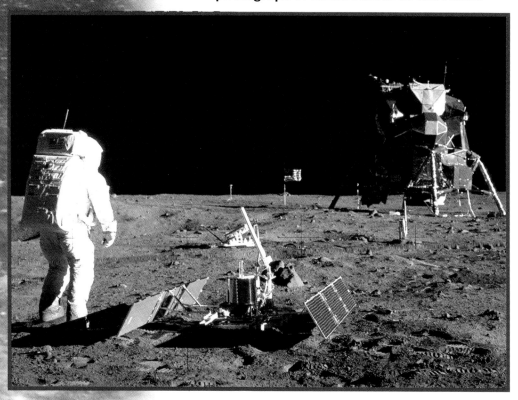

The second lunar landing mission, Apollo 12, was a 10-day mission during which the crew spent more than 7 hours exploring the surface of the Moon. At the end of this mission, the spacecraft once again landed safely in the Pacific Ocean.

The third planned lunar landing was Apollo 13. Two days after it launched, an explosion took place and the astronauts had to return to Earth unexpectedly. The crew on the ground had to work quickly with the astronauts to help get them safely back to Earth.

James A. Lovell, the mission commander, was in charge of figuring out a new flight plan. He and dozens of scientists had to recalculate the original flight plan numbers to get the spacecraft back to Earth safely under emergency conditions.

At one point in the mission, Lovell had to find the craft's position by adding and subtracting numbers from the navigation system. The calculations were so important that Lovell asked the crew on the ground to check his arithmetic. Luckily, his math was correct, and the spacecraft was able to return safely to Earth.

The Need for Speed

Because space is so big, space travel requires some very fast and powerful spacecraft for getting around. Without these spacecraft it would take a very long time to get anywhere in space.

For instance, imagine if a jet could fly from the Earth to the Sun. If the jet traveled at 600 miles per hour, it would still take 18 years to get there.

The Apollo Missions

During the Apollo missions to the Moon, a rocket was developed that was powerful enough to reach the Moon. The craft got to the Moon and then was able to travel back to Earth.

One spacecraft that is used to get to space quickly is the space shuttle. To reach space, the shuttle can **accelerate** to almost 18,000 miles per hour!

The shuttle's two solid rocket boosters fire and help the shuttle's three main engines push the shuttle up during launch. By the time the shuttle has traveled for 8 seconds, it has accelerated to 100 miles per hour. After the first minute, it reaches more than 1,000 miles per hour. After about 2 minutes, the shuttle speeds along at 3,000 miles per hour. Once it reaches 150 miles above Earth, the shuttle cruises at almost 18,000 miles per hour.

The space shuttle starts at 0 and reaches 1,000 miles per hour just 1 minute after launch.

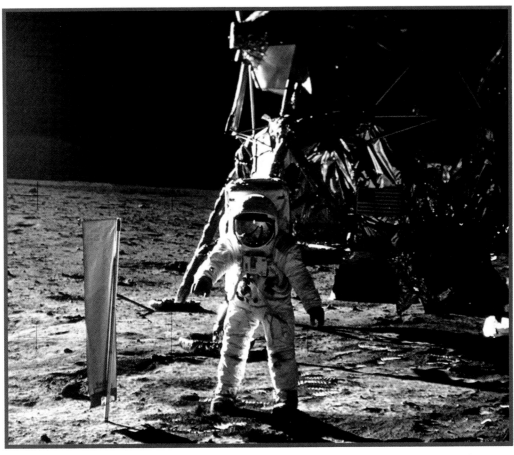

This astronaut—Edwin Aldrin—reached the Moon in an Apollo spacecraft. His landing craft, the *Eagle*, is behind him.

The space shuttle isn't designed to go to the Moon. It's made to travel to the International Space Station or to orbit, which means "to circle the Earth in space." If it could go to the Moon, it could get there in half a day. That's if it traveled at its top speed the whole way.

More than 35 years ago, it took astronauts 2 days to reach the Moon. They used the pull of the Moon to help tug their spaceship. On the way home, they used the pull of the Earth's gravity to travel back.

Gravity is a force that has to be considered in all space missions. It is not only a force on Earth. Every planet has its own gravity. On each planet, the gravity is different.

Gravity is determined by the mass of a planet, that is, how much matter it contains. Therefore, larger planets have more gravity and smaller planets have less gravity. We measure gravity on a scale: Your weight is the measure of gravity's pull on you. If you were to travel to another planet, your weight would be different.

What would you weigh?

Say you weigh 100 pounds on Earth. Here is what you would weigh on:

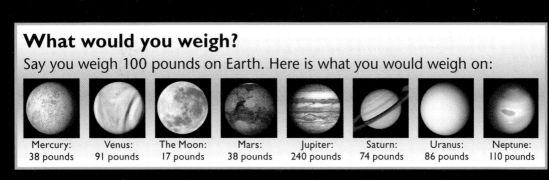

Mercury:	Venus:	The Moon:	Mars:	Jupiter:	Saturn:	Uranus:	Neptune:
38 pounds	91 pounds	17 pounds	38 pounds	240 pounds	74 pounds	86 pounds	110 pounds

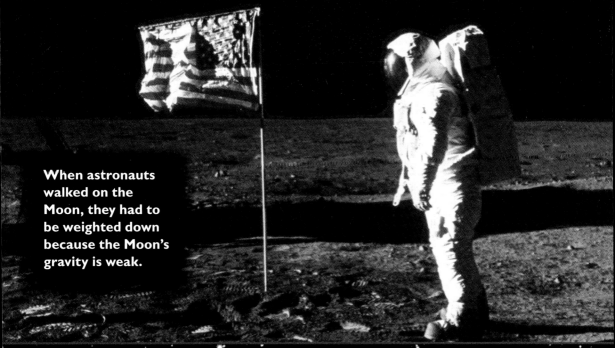

When astronauts walked on the Moon, they had to be weighted down because the Moon's gravity is weak.

Planning a Space Mission

Speed and gravity aren't the only things scientists have to consider when sending crafts into space. They also have to time a launch so a spacecraft can reach its destination. Sometimes this means the spacecraft has a very limited time when it can launch. The time the spacecraft can set off is known as the **launch window**. The launch window depends on factors such as lighting and weather, as well as other conditions in space. It takes many calculations to figure out the launch window.

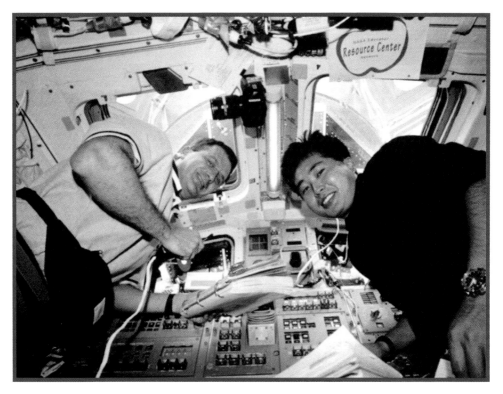

Space scientists have to do many kinds of calculations.

Think about a trip to the International Space Station. The space station is a base that astronauts built in space. Like the Moon, the space station constantly orbits Earth. When the space shuttle reaches space, it also orbits Earth. When scientists want to send the space shuttle to the space station, they have to time it just right so the orbits of the space shuttle and the space station meet up. That means a launch needs to happen at just the right time.

a view of the space shuttle docked at the International Space Station with Earth below

Mission planners also have to think about the weather when they make their calculations. The weather has to be good when the space shuttle launches and when it lands. That requires looking ahead to the space shuttle's landing date. There are so many factors to take into account that planning a space mission can seem like juggling. It also means that the space shuttle's launch window can be very small.

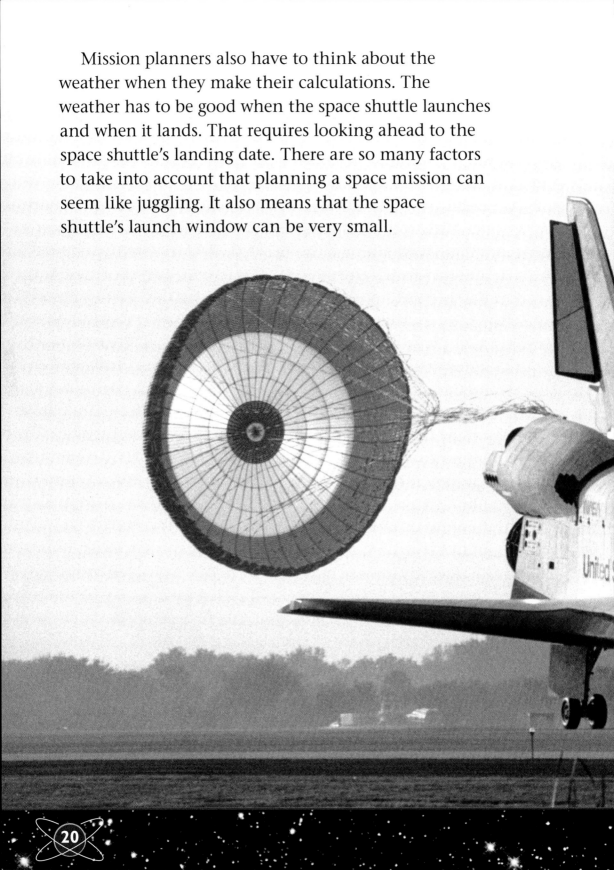

Imagine the work of an engineer for NASA who has to decide when the space shuttle should launch. Consider how many things need to be calculated. Here is an example of what might go into the calculations.

Say the spaceship is supposed to land at the space station and return to Earth in 12 days. It takes 2 days from launch to meet up with the station. The space shuttle must launch between 10 a.m. and 10:20 a.m. to make sure its orbit matches with the station's. That's when they'll both be at the same points in space.

Most space shuttles land on a 3-mile runway at the Kennedy Space Center.

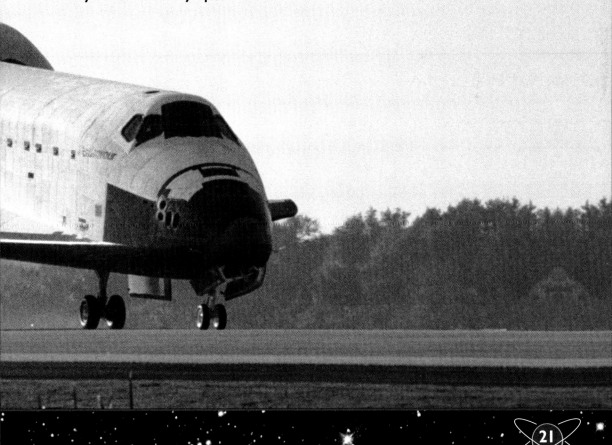

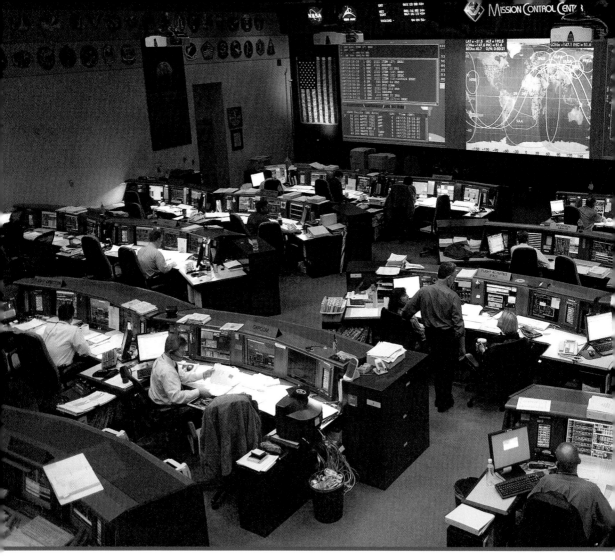

Mission planners have to do many calculations to decide when to launch.

The weather for launch day looks good—except after 4 p.m., when winds will become strong. The weather in 12 days looks good for landing only for 3 hours, from 11 a.m. to 2 p.m. To set the launch time, NASA engineers must keep all these things in mind. If conditions change, they have to adjust their calculations.

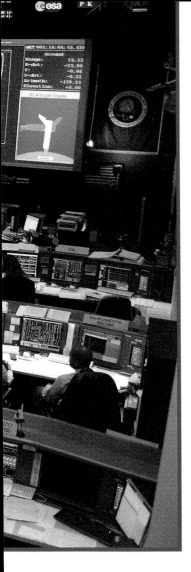

Metric Matters

Most scientists use the metric system. The system was developed in France in the 1790s. It is based on powers of ten.

The metric system uses the meter (which is about the same length as a yard) as the base unit for length. Both the kilometer and the **millimeter** are based on the meter.

To measure a longer length, you use the kilometer, which is 1,000 times the length of a meter. Smaller lengths can be measured with the centimeter, which is $\frac{1}{100}$ the length of a meter. A very small length would be measured with the millimeter, which is $\frac{1}{1,000}$ the length of a meter.

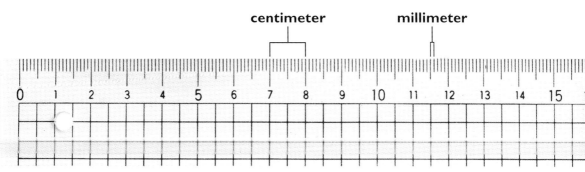

a metric ruler

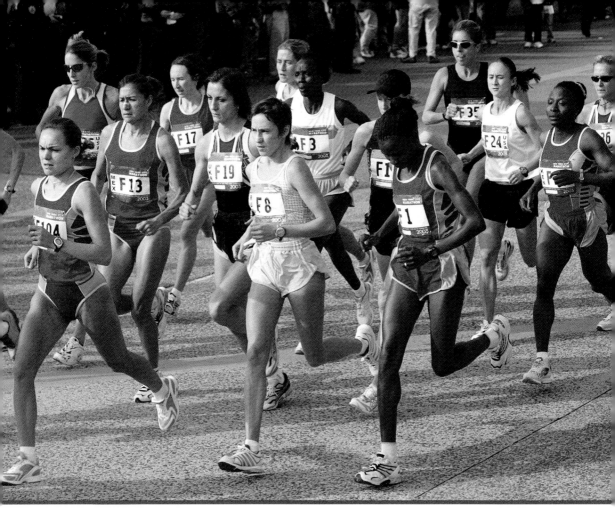

Many track events in the United States measure races in yards and miles. These distances are from the English system of measurement.

People in the United States often use a different kind of measurement system known as the English system. Units in the English system are based on old measurements first used in England. Most scientists don't use English units because they don't share a common base like the metric system. Instead of one base unit to measure distance, the English system has inches, feet, yards, and miles. That can make calculations confusing.

A Costly Mistake

In 1999, NASA scientists tried to land a spacecraft on Mars. The spacecraft, called the *Mars Climate Orbiter*, cost $125 million to build. It traveled for 286 days and got within 60 miles of Mars. Then, on September 23, 1999, it was lost. What happened?

When people looked into what may have gone wrong, they were shocked. One team of planners used English units while another used the metric system. Calculations from both teams were fed into the spacecraft's computer.

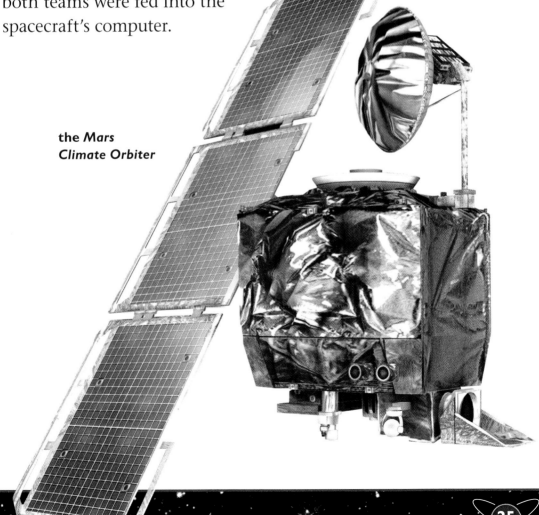

the *Mars Climate Orbiter*

Because their calculations were based on different measuring systems, the spacecraft received conflicting instructions and became "confused." The spacecraft got too close to Mars before preparing to go into orbit. Then it overheated and probably burned up in the atmosphere of Mars. If both teams had used the metric system, the spacecraft would have moved safely into orbit around Mars. That expensive error taught planners a lesson: From then on, everyone had to use the same system, and the metric system was chosen.

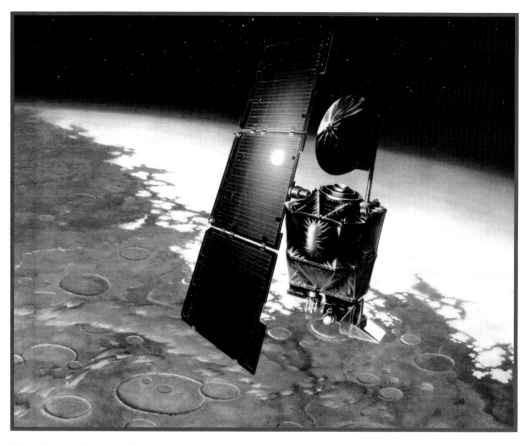

The *Mars Climate Orbiter* was lost when scientists used different kinds of measurements to plan its journey.

Going Farther and Deeper

Losing the *Mars Climate Orbiter* showed how hard it is to send a spacecraft into space. In fact, scientists lost another spacecraft, the *Mars Polar Lander*, on its way to Mars just 3 months later. Again, it seems a mistake in calculations was probably the cause. The craft turned off its descent engines too soon as it was landing, and it crashed into the planet.

There are so many calculations that go into a space mission that making one little mistake can ruin an entire mission. Mars is such a long way away from Earth that getting things there is very challenging. Now, imagine sending a spacecraft even farther away.

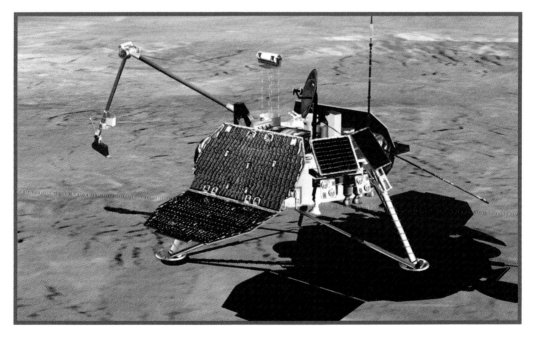

The *Mars Polar Lander* was lost attempting to land on Mars.

There are entire star systems in space other than our own solar system. The nearest star system is Alpha Centauri. The nearest star in it is Proxima Centauri, which is about 4.2 light-years away. A light-year is the distance light would travel in 1 year.

The fastest thing scientists know of in space is light. It travels about 186,000 miles per second. In 1 year, light travels about 5.88 trillion miles. Since Proxima Centauri is about 4.2 light-years away, that means our nearest neighboring star is 25 trillion miles away! One trillion is equal to 1,000 times 1,000,000,000. That's 1,000,000,000,000, or one million million.

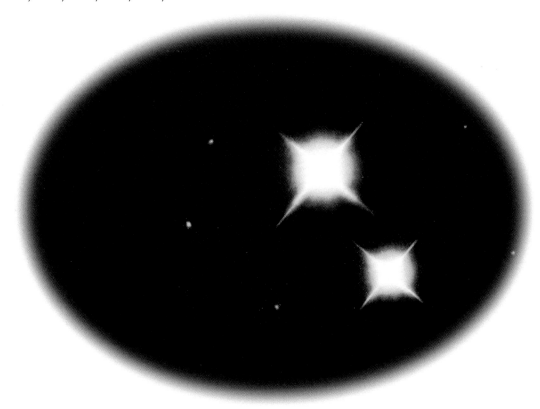

Proxima Centauri is the nearest star, but it is still 25 trillion miles away!

Looking at light from distant solar systems is the same as looking back in time.

Think about how long it would take the space shuttle to reach the nearest solar system. Even if the shuttle traveled at top speed the whole way, it would still take a very long time. Getting to the nearest solar system would take more than 162,000 years. The fact is, we just can't travel fast enough yet to go great distances in space.

Even seeing distant objects in space is tricky. Stars in other systems are so far away that it can take millions of years for their light to reach Earth. By the time people on Earth see their light, the stars may no longer exist.

Math can help scientists to understand space and how to explore it. It can help scientists look into the past and better understand how the past affects the present and the future. For example, if a person sees light from a star that's 50 light-years away, what is that person seeing? Calculations show the person is actually looking back in time by 50 years!

Maybe someday people will be able to travel farther into space and see greater distances. In the meantime, math offers scientists a tool to explore what lies beyond their reach.

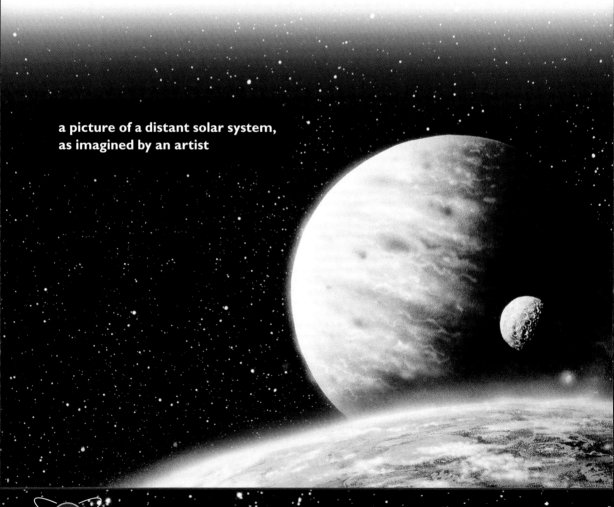

a picture of a distant solar system, as imagined by an artist

Glossary

accelerate   to move faster

calculations   results found by using math

kilometers   measures of length; 1 kilometer is equal to 1,000 meters or 3,280.84 feet

lasers   instruments that send out intense, directed beams of light

launch window   the time that a spacecraft can launch while meeting its goals and staying within safety guidelines

millimeter   a measure of length that is equal to 0.001 of a meter or 0.0394 of an inch

precisely   exactly

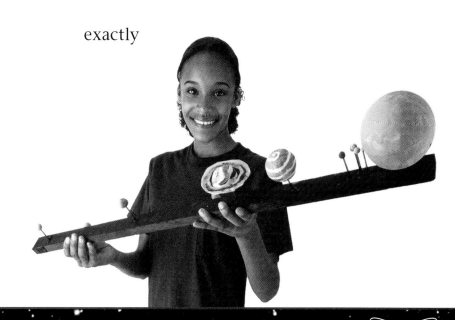

Index

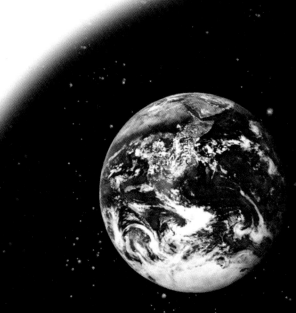